ENDOBRONCHIAL ULTRASOUND and EBUS-GUIDED TBNA

TRAINING MANUAL

SECOND EDITION

HENRI G COLT M.D. FAWM, FCCP

BRONCHOSCOPY INTERNATIONAL

BRONCHOSCOPY INTERNATIONAL

THE BRONCHOSCOPY EDUCATION PROJECT SERIES

rake press

THE BRONCHOSCOPY EDUCATION PROJECT SERIES

SECOND EDITION

Henri G. Colt MD, FAWM, FCCP

This Second Edition of **The Bronchoscopy Education Project Series** of training manuals constitutes part of the highly regarded Bronchoscopy Education Project. These training manuals provide a broad perspective on the art, knowledge, science, and technical skills that must be acquired in order to be a competent bronchoscopist. They are written for bronchoscopy educators and all those who wish to improve upon their ability to teach and mentor bronchoscopists regardless of specialty. Of course, readers are encouraged to also study, *The Essential Bronchoscopist© Series* of learning materials and to participate in our many Faculty Development (train-the-Trainer) programs conducted all over the world in collaboration with many national bronchology and interventional associations.

Each **Training Manual** incorporates theories and instructional modalities as part of our competency-oriented training and mastery learning philosophies. Educational modalities are learner-centric, always emphasizing that the end result must be patient-driven.

Each volume in the series pertains to a different aspect of bronchoscopic practice. The overall structure of each volume, however, is similar, containing examples of on-site course agendas, a summary of reading materials, selected references, a description of step-by-step technical skill instruction, simulation workshop scenarios, patient-based practical approach exercises, validated assessment tools to monitor progress along the learning curve, and a series of checklists designed to enhance patient, operator, and equipment safety. Patients must no longer suffer the burden of physician learning.

Readers are encouraged to download additional materials from our website (www.bronchoscopy.org) and view instructional videos from the BronchOrg YouTube channel and other sources as well as attend regional seminars and participate in apprentice-like training experiences. With your help and the support of national organizations and associations such as the *World Association for Bronchology and Interventional Pulmonology*, **The Bronchoscopy Education Project** can help bring uniformity to medical procedural training for years to come.

Training Manuals

- INTRODUCTION TO FLEXIBLE BRONCHOSCOPY
- ENDOBRONCHIAL ULTRASOUND AND EBUS-GUIDED TBNA
- LEARNING AND TEACHING BRONCHOSCOPY

BRONCHOSCOPY INTERNATIONAL

Sponsored by Bronchoscopy International, Laguna Beach, CA 92651

Colt Henri G

Endobronchial Ultrasound and EBUS-Guided TBNA Training Manual Bronchoscopy Education Project Series of Training Manuals

ISBN 978-0-9848347-2-3
Endobronchial Ultrasound and EBUS-Guided TBNA

1. Colt HG, 1956-

Publisher Rake Press
Laguna Beach, CA

Manufactured in the United States of America

1 2 3 4 5 6 7 8 9 10

rake
press

THE BRONCHOSCOPY EDUCATION PROJECT SERIES

ENDOBRONCHIAL ULTRASOUND And EBUS-GUIDED TBNA

TRAINING MANUAL

SECOND EDITION

HENRI G COLT MD, FAWM, FCCP

BRONCHOSCOPY INTERNATIONAL

With contributions from Drs S. Murgu, E. Edell, S. Quadrelli, and M. Davoudi, and J. Williamson.

Notice: Knowledge changes. We have done our best to assure references to procedures, medications, and techniques are correct and compatible with standards of practice at the time of publication. We are proud that Checklists, Assessment tools, and Bronchoscopy Step-by-Step instructional methods are commonly used around the world. Future editions may include modifications based on user feedback and new information. Any doctor, patient, or hospital names used in simulation/learning scenarios in this manual are fictitious.

Distributed by Bronchoscopy International*, The World Association for Bronchology and Interventional Pulmonology, and national bronchology and interventional pulmonology societies.

rake press

Printed in the United States

* Bronchoscopy International Foundation for the Advancement of Medicine; a 501c3 Non-Profit Foundation Registry # 33-0593357

ACKNOWLEDGMENTS

This Bronchoscopy Education Project training manual could not have been written without the help and advice of numerous colleagues from around the world who enthusiastically use the training modalities described herein. These regional champions are changing the paradigm of procedure-related learning to the great benefit of our patients and society. Their confidence in the process is particularly inspiring in the face of resistance from established practitioners who advocate a more conventional manner of instruction. Of course, my thanks also to patients everywhere who without questions have until recently suffered the burden of procedure-related training at the hands of health care professionals who learn solely by doing.

ABOUT THE AUTHOR

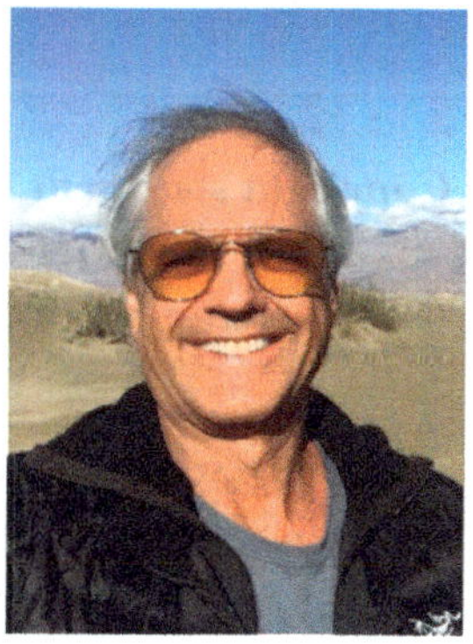

HENRI COLT is an award-winning medical educator, ethicist and philosophical practitioner. In addition to authoring scientific papers and several medical textbooks, he is the author/editor of the popular *The Picture of Health: Medical Ethics and the Movies* (Oxford University Press) and nonfiction works such as *Modigliani: Art & illness.* His *Essential Bronchoscopist* series of books and medical training tools have been translated into 14 languages. His *Bronchoscopy and Central Airway Disorders: A Patient-centered Approach* (Elsevier press) with coauthor Professor Septimiu Murgu is a textbook standard for Interventional pulmonologists and airway specialists around the world.

Dr. Colt is University of California Emeritus Professor of Pulmonary and Critical Care Medicine. When he is not traveling, writing or teaching, he is dancing tango or climbing mountains in far away places.

Funding statement

Funding for The Bronchoscopy Education Project Series is a result of philanthropic endeavors No corporate support was either solicited or received for this work.

Bronchoscopy International is a transnational group of volunteers working under the auspices of The Foundation for the Advancement of Medicine, a 501-C3 non-profit organization registered in San Diego, CA, USA (Registry # 33-0593357).

Bronchoscopy Education Project Disclaimer

Confidentiality of data potentially relating to individual patients has been respected. We strive to honor or exceed any legal requirements of medical/health information privacy as they apply to the United States and to the state of California.

Images and case descriptions provided here-in, therefore, are not intended for the diagnosis of any specific patient. Any information found on the website or in this text should not be used as a substitute for medical care.

The authors disclaim liability, injury, or damage incurred as a consequence from the use of information. Reference to websites, instruments, or equipment portrayed in this material is not of commercial nature, nor does the inclusion imply endorsement.

Should documents or images from this material be copied for personal use, we request that materials remain unedited and unmodified unless for teaching purposes, that no fee be charged for copies or access to the information, that copyright notices and disclaimers remain attached, and that credit be given to The Bronchoscopy Education Project (suggested format Bronchoscopy International® www.bronchoscopy.org).

rake press

Table of Contents

WELCOME
to the
Bronchoscopy Education Project

This collection of competency-oriented tools and materials was designed with a philosophy of mastery training in mind. Competency is the minimum threshold acceptable for medical procedural practice. Bronchoscopy International is a collegial group of expert bronchoscopist-educators devoted to teaching using a paradigm in which patients never suffer the burden of procedure-related learning. While the learner-centric structure of the project targets bronchoscopy, it is readily applied to other procedural areas of medical training.

Part II of **The Bronchoscopy Education Project** is an **Endobronchial Ultrasound and (convex probe)**[i] **EBUS-Guided TBNA©.** This competency program addresses course organization, ultrasound physics, EBUS equipment and instrumentation, mediastinal exploration and staging, radiographic-bronchoscopic correlations, image analysis, tumor markers, specimen handling, team dynamics and communication, and EBUS-related techniques This training manual can be used with **The Essential EBUS Bronchoscopist©,** a compilation of thirty question/answer sets pertaining to convex probe endobronchial ultrasound and EBUS-Guided Transbronchial Needle Aspiration (TBNA).

Materials from the Bronchoscopy Education Project can be incorporated in whole or in part into training programs. Other learning and teaching materials are available at our website, www.bronchoscopy.org. Welcome to the exciting world of Bronchoscopy Education. We look forward to your comments as you use these materials.

Henri Colt MD., FAWM, FCCP
henricolt@Bronchoscopy.org

The Shifting Paradigm of Bronchoscopy Education

Halstedt's model of graduate medical education based on a see one, do one, teach one paradigm implemented in the last century has been the traditional method of acquired learning during medical apprenticeship. Its relevance has come into question because this educational model is adversely affected by constraints of training for a fixed period of time, the presumed need to assimilate material through formal didactic and on-site teachings, a lack of alternatives to learning on patients, a tendency towards variability[1,2], and a presumption that learning curves are climbed by performing a minimum number of procedures while assuming an escalating number of responsibilities during training. In the absence of competency-oriented examinations, currently written exams and numbers requirements for procedures still provide some objective criteria on which to base competency[3].

The paradigm shift in bronchoscopy education has now occurred[4]. It is simply a matter of time and education that teachers and mentors all over the world implement new educational programs and methodologies. The diversity of medical practice and training is now recognized, and already accounts for changing constructs of training curricula[5]. Time and cost restraints prompt physicians to find ways with which to incorporate teaching and procedure-related training into a more effective and efficient clinical practice (Figure 1, abstracted from reference 4). Teaching is increasingly separated from clinical service responsibilities, and educators are using competency-oriented tools rather than subjective assessments and "observed experience" to enhance training. Information is increasingly accessible through social media and electronic media libraries. Literature searches of peer reviewed journals and other publications are at the students' fingertips.

Furthermore, universities and professional societies provide web-based instruction and continued medical education so learners can study materials at their own pace and according to their own busy schedules. Flipped classroom techniques are being used to improve and workshop one-on-one practical performance sessions, and the proven value of inanimate model and computer-based simulation, in addition to the recognized effectiveness of patient surrogates, problem-based learning, and practice-based interactive sessions render experiential learning based solely on patient encounters increasingly obsolete. Finally, has become evident that neither patients nor their novice physicians should be submitted to the potentially unethical practice of learning by doing, especially early in the course of training.

In the following paragraphs we describe several elements of a bronchoscopy educational program based on the premise that patients not bear the burden of procedure-related training. While we focus on the art and practice of flexible bronchoscopy, we propose that similar curricular structure are applicable to all fields of procedural medical practice. A social mandate for effective, efficient, safe, and ethically responsible clinical care warrants that we reassess older educational methodologies, and that we incorporate new techniques into the learning process. These techniques can often be individualized according to a learner's needs, and may enhance an accelerated climb of a procedural learning curve, assist in imparting knowledge to learners outside of the patient practice setting, avoid many of the shortcomings of existing and well-recognized variations in medical training, and allow the design of a more structured, uniform competency-oriented curriculum that can be individually tailored to fill the needs of diverse practices, cultures, and medical environments[6].

In general, procedure-based education requires factual knowledge, technical skill, experience, and a recognition of the effect of patient-procedural interactions on personal affectivity[i]. *Knowledge* generally refers to the acquisition of information required by a physician to make a medical decision. In this regard, cognitive knowledge refers to studies of cognitive processes such as perception, comprehension, decision-making and problem-solving that affect the decision-making process, whereas medical reasoning might apply to the acquisition of a series of skills that enable a clinical decision[ii].

Assessments are often used to identify what and how much learners are learning, how well they are progressing in their acquisition of knowledge and skills, their position on the learning curve, and to help identify the strengths and weaknesses of a curriculum. A combination of low and high-stakes testing might be used to provide opportunities for bidirectional feedback, need for remedial intervention, establish criteria for competency or modify certain elements of curricular structure if learners' needs are not being sufficiently addressed[7]. High-stakes assessments usually entail a pass-fail threshold with significant consequences for the learner, whereas low-stakes assessments are often performed as part of a curriculum to judge progress in the acquisition of knowledge or skill. A competency-based educational curriculum, therefore, must include elements that are teachable, learnable and measurable. Hence, *competence* is defined as the verifiable assimilation of a specific set of knowledge, skills, behaviors, attitudes, and educational experiences required of trainees to complete such graduate medical education programs[8,9,10,11].

The bronchoscopy-related literature supports the paradigm shift whereby patients will no longer bear the burden of procedure-related training. In a review of several papers pertaining to the use of simulation for bronchoscopy education[12], simulation was demonstrated to help learners improve procedural efficiency and economy of movement, thoroughness and accuracy of airway examination, and incidence of airway wall trauma. Both lo- and hi-fidelity simulation have been shown to enhance physician competency in procedural skills, while saving time and accelerating a learner's ascent of the learning curve. Hi-fidelity simulation platforms using three-dimensional virtual anatomy and force feedback technology can be used to learn bronchoscopic inspection, biopsy, brushing, conventional transbronchial needle aspiration and convex-probe endobronchial ultrasound-guided-TBNA, although less expensive, lo-fidelity models comprised of molded silicone or excised animal airways, are also very effective[13,14,15,16,17]. In the last ten years, results from numerous studies show the many benefits of simulation-based training.

In addition to increasing learner satisfaction and interest, simulated environments and structured curricular learning create opportunities where the uniformization of information is enhanced, tasks can be practiced repeatedly, risks to patients are eliminated, and training scenarios can be tailored to individual

---

[i] How one perceives the experience and responds to situations from an emotional, psychological and behavioral perspective. This is different from experiential learning, which, for example, might entail one's accumulation of knowledge based on a series of similar cases.

[ii] For example, the knowledge of and ability to apply clinical pathways or algorithms, and justify one's diversion from an algorithmic pathway in certain circumstances.

learners' needs. Procedural skills acquired through practice on simulators are considered transferable to the clinical setting (Figure 2), and objective assessments performed at time of training helps identify errors and provides opportunities for repeated, focused practice without exposing patients to the discomfort of unnecessarily prolonged procedures. Reading assignments should probably be mandatory to assure compliance[18], and validated assessment tools can be incorporated into learning curricula to help identify acquisition of knowledge and skills[19], as well as to study the effectiveness of a learning program[iii].

In an attempt to provide a curriculum that might be widely available and broadly applicable in diverse medical cultures and practice environments, a six-part program was designed to be accessed, in part, via the Internet, but also incorporated in whole or in part into continued medical education postgraduate seminars or formal institution-based training programs. This program includes reading material, a growing pictorial and video atlas, a step-by-step exercise-based technique for learning bronchoscopic inspection, a series of didactic and interactive lectures pertaining to the art and science of bronchoscopy, an assortment of patient-centered practical approach exercises to assist with acquiring the knowledge and skills required for appropriate procedure-related medical decision-making, and a group of validated assessment and self-assessment tools[iv]. Many of these materials are available on the Bronchoscopy International website (www.Bronchoscopy.org)[v]. Instructional videos are accessible on the website as well as directly on the Bronchoscopy International You Tube and Facebook pages.

In order to further disseminate and eventually study the impact of these methodologies from an educational research perspective, the curriculum has been incorporated into the **Bronchoscopy Education Project**. The purpose of this project is to provide educators, training program directors, and bronchoscopists in practice or in-training with competency-oriented tools and materials that can be used to assess progression along the learning curve from novice to competent practitioner. The uniform curriculum is built on a template that includes course schedules, informational content[20], checklists[vi], validated assessment tools, description and use of training models, simulation scenarios, patient-centered practical approach exercises, and a series of didactic and interactive lectures[21].

The BEP has been officially endorsed by numerous national bronchology and interventional pulmonology organizations, as well as by the AABIP, EABIP, WABIP, and the ASER[vii]. Some of the original practical investigations of several elements from this curriculum were undertaken with the help of the Argentine Association for Bronchology and Esophagology and The Singapore Thoracic Society. Faculty development programs are ongoing to help educators assimilate assorted techniques, implement educational methodologies,

---

[iii] Such as one that includes a one or two-day program of didactic lectures, hands-on learning, and interactive case-based scenarios. Class-average normalized gain (in addition to the calculation of absolute and relative gain) can be particularly helpful in this regard. (g) is defined as the average actual gain divided by the maximum possible gain (see Colt HG, et al., Surg Endosc 2011;25:207-216, available from the authors on request)

[iv] For example, The Essential Bronchoscopist© now translated into nine languages, the EBUS Bronchoscopist©, BronchAtlas™, the Art of Bronchoscopy©, Bronchoscopy Step-by-Step©, Practical Approach to Procedural Decision-Making, and Bronchoscopy Assessment Tools© (Bronchoscopy Skills and Tasks© [BSTAT], Bronchoscopy Self- Assessment Tool [BSAT], and Endobronchial Ultrasound Skills and Tasks© [EBUS-STAT].

[v] Bronchoscopy International is a no hierarchal group of motivated bronchoscopy educators serving as an integrated part of the 501-C3 non-profit Foundation for the Advancement of Medicine.

[vi] Examples of Checklists include Fluoroscopy, Informed Consent, Procedural pause, Moderate sedation, Practical approach, Proctored flexible bronchoscopy, and Program completion.

[vii] Abbreviations for American Association for Bronchology and Interventional Pulmonology, European Association for Bronchology and Interventional Pulmonology, World Association for Bronchology and Interventional Pulmonology, Asociaccion Sudamericana Endoscopia Respiratoria

master the application of the various assessment tools, practice their delivery of didactic lectures, and facilitate of interactive sessions. Programs provide opportunities for self-assessment, acquisition of debriefing skills and 360-degree feedback to enhance teaching skills[22,23]. These programs are made available through the generous support and assistance of international volunteer faculty, training institutions, and national or international societies, with the addition of material support for hands-on learning stations provided from equipment manufacturers and the World Association for Bronchology and Interventional Pulmonology.

We believe interventional pulmonary procedures such as bronchoscopy are performed more competently by bronchoscopists who possess a uniform foundation of theoretic knowledge and standardized skill. The uniformization of educational content and process has the potential to facilitate social interactions, knowledge transfer, and equality of care regardless of one's medical practice environment. The paradigm shift in bronchoscopy education, however, should not be taken lightly. Curricular content needs to be regularly revised and new assessment tools will require validation in specific target settings. Philosophies of competency-oriented training and mastery learning are not easily adopted without significant effort, and more research is warranted to assess their effectiveness.

Figure 1: Educational methodologies. From, Colt HG and Williamson J Respirology. 2020 25(9):997-1007.

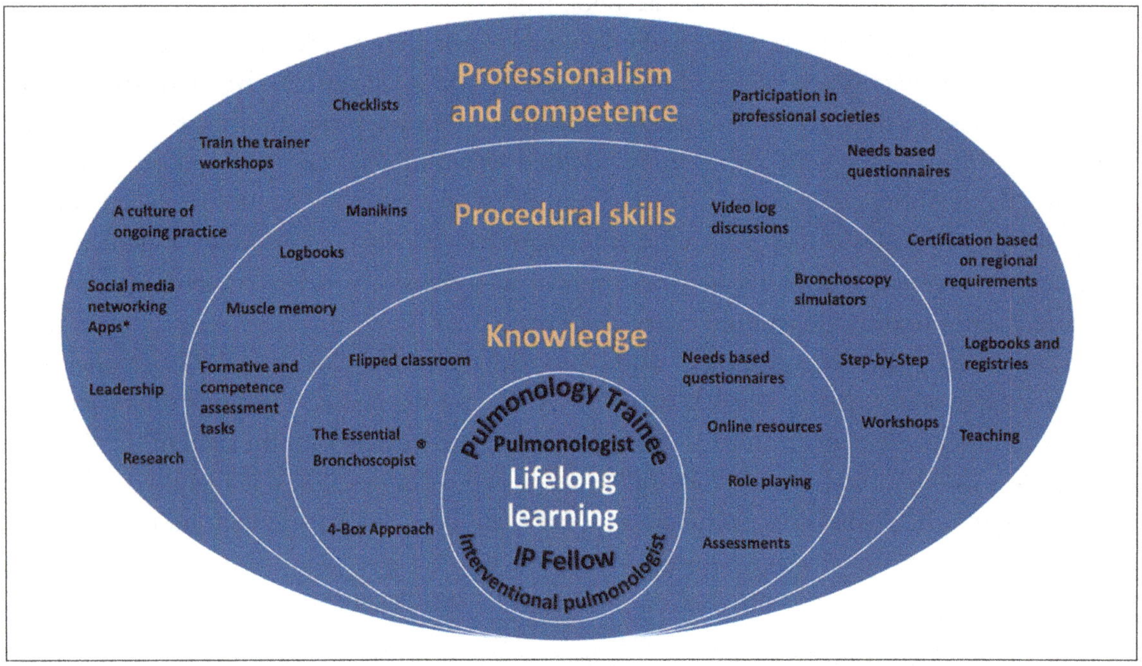

Figure 2: Examples of inanimate and computer-based simulation models for learning flexible bronchoscopy.

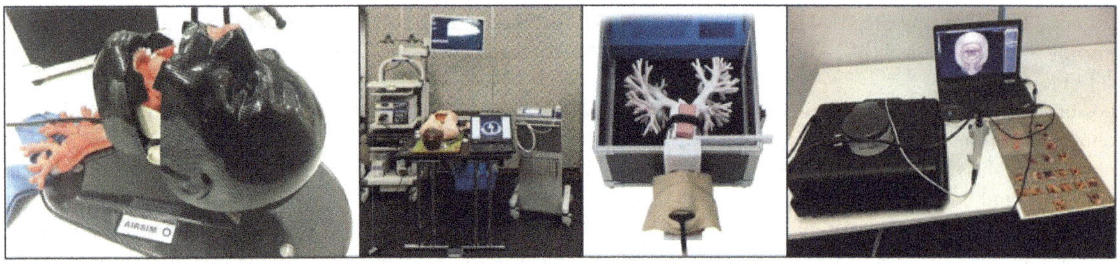

References

1. Pastis N, Silvestri, G et al. ACCP interventional chest diagnostic procedures network steering committee. Variation in training for interventional pulmonary procedures among US pulmonary critical care fellowships, a survey of Fellowship directors. Chest. 2005; 127:1614 – 1621.
2. Pyng L, Loo CM, Jagadesan R, Colt HG. Survey of bronchoscopy practice in Singapore. J Bronchol 2008;15(4):215-220.
3. Torrington KG. Bronchoscopy training and competency: How many are enough? Chest 1999;118:572-573.
4. Colt HG, Williamson JP. Training in interventional pulmonology: What we have learned and a way forward. Respirology. 2020 Sep;25(9):997-1007. doi: 10.1111/resp.13846. Epub 2020 May 26. PMID: 32453479.
5. Haponik EF, Russell GB, Beamis JF, et al. Bronchoscopy training: Current fellows, experiences, and some concerns for the future. Chest. 2000; 118:572 – 573.
6. Long DM. Competency based residency training: the next advance in graduate medical education. Academic Medicine 2000;75(12):1178-1183.
7. Quadrelli S, Galíndez F, Davoudi M Colt HG. Reliability of a 25 item *low stakes* multiple choice assessment of bronchoscopic knowledge. Chest 2009;135:315-321.
8. Marinopoulos SS, Baumann MH. Methods and definitions of terms: effectiveness of continuing medical education: American College of Chest Physicians evidence-based educational guidelines. Chest 2009;135:17S–28S.
9. Patel VL, Aroca JF, and Zhang J. Thinking, and reasoning in medicine. In The Cambridge handbook of thinking and reasoning. KJ Holyoake & Morrison RG Editors. University Press, Cambridge UK 2005.
10. High stakes testing "http://en.wikipedia.org/wiki/High-stakes testing". Retrieved on March 20, 2008.
11. Miller GE. The assessment of clinical skills, competence and performance. Academic medicine 1990;65 (9 supplements): S63–7.
12. Davoudi M, Colt HG. Bronchoscopy simulation: a brief review. Adv Health Sci Educ 2009;14:287-296.
13. Davoudi M, Wahidi MM, Rohani NZ, Colt HG. Comparative effectiveness of low and high-fidelity bronchoscopy simulation for training in conventional transbronchial needle aspiration and user preferences. Respiration 2010;80:327-334.
14. Ost D, DeRosiers A, Britt EJ, et al. Assessment of a bronchoscopy simulator. Am J Respir Crit Care Med 2001;164(12):2248-55.
15. Crawford SW and Colt HG. Virtual reality and written assessments are of potential value to determine knowledge and skill in flexible bronchoscopy. Respiration 2004; 71:269 – 275.
16. Colt HG, Crawford, SW., Galbraith O. Virtual reality bronchoscopy simulation: A revolution in procedural training. Chest 2001; 120(4):1333–1339.
17. Goldberg R, Colt HG, Davoudi M, Cherisson L. Realistic and affordable lo-fidelity model for learning transbronchial needle aspiration. Surg Endosc;2009 Sep; 23(9): 2047-52.
18. Wahidi MM, Silvestri GA, Coakley RD, Ferguson JS, Shepherd RW, Moses L, Conforti. J, Que L, Anstrom KJ, McGuire F, Colt H, Downie GH. A prospective multi-center study of competency metrics and educational interventions in the learning of bronchoscopy among starting pulmonary fellows. Chest 2010;137(5):1040-1049.
19. Davoudi M, Osann K, and Colt HG. Validation of two instruments to assess technical bronchoscopy skill using virtual reality simulation. Respiration 2008;76:92-101.
20. Davoudi M, Quadrelli S, Osann K, and Colt HG. A competency-based test of bronchoscopic knowledge using the Essential Bronchoscopist: an initial concept study. Respirology 2008;13:736-743.
21. Colt HG, Davoudi M, Murgu S, and Rohani NZ. Measuring learning gain during a one-day introductory bronchoscopy course. Surg Endoscopy 2010;25:207-216.
22. Rudolph JW, Simon R, Dufresne RL, et al. There's no such thing as nonjudgemental debriefing. A theory and method for debriefing with good judgement. Simulation in Healthcare 2006;1:49-55.
23. Goldsmith M and Underhill B. 2001. Multisource feedback for executive development. In D. Bracken, C Timmreck and A. Church (eds). The handbook of multi-source feedback, pp 275-288. Jossey-Bass: San Francisco.

****

Training in Interventional Pulmonology: New ways forward

Extracted in part from: Colt HG, Williamson JP. Training in interventional pulmonology: What we have learned and a way forward. Respirology. 2020 Sep;25(9):997-1007. doi: 10.1111/resp.13846. Epub 2020 May 26. PMID: 32453479.

Until recently, training strategies for Interventional pulmonology (IP) were intrinsically linked to the see one, do one, teach one apprentice-style model traditionally used for centuries in medical education. Teaching methodologies were patriarchal in nature, often reflecting power differentials between teacher and learner, as well as hierarchal structures and the idea that it is was permissible to use patients as a basis for learning.

Thankfully, times are changing. According to data from the Association of American Medical Colleges, medical schools in the United States are increasingly diverse, and women now make up more than 50% of classes, a trend also found in many other countries[1]. Furthermore, increased familiarity with social media and the internet makes sharing information and experience instantaneous. New educational paradigms focused on the democratization of knowledge encourage access to these technologies, as well as to using inanimate models and computer-based simulation rather than patients to practice and perfect procedural skills. These methods allow independent learning with a focus on objective measures of competence using specifically-designed assessment tools that are now accepted, not only for measuring technical skills, but also for demonstrating skills with problem-solving, differential diagnosis, informed consent and other components of the medical encounter.

Radical, disruptive, and transformative changes do not occur without challenges. People and institutions are reluctant to abandon traditional ways of thinking and slow to adapt to new paradigms. This natural resistance, coupled with the accelerating speed of technological evolution and conflicts faced in teaching environments where optimal patient care must be balanced with cost concerns, time-efficiency, expectations for quality, safety, and accountability, as well as with an instructor's goal to impart knowledge and the trainee's desire to master skills essential to their careers, provides a situational background that is common to many countries.

Indeed, the nature of interventional pulmonology suggests that training programs should provide learners with a broad exposure to more than just technical skills. Opportunities to assess the acquisition of many forms of knowledge, including those needed to nurture humanistic qualities and medical expertise are also desirable. Of course, there is a minimum requirement for practitioners is to dedicate time and energy to learning bronchoscopy and other interventional procedures under the guidance of experts. The increasing number of possible interventions, in addition to decreased durations of hospitalizations, a limited source of patients, overwhelming amounts of information and procedure-related technologies, and rising health care costs makes it essential for anyone learning procedures to master what some might call basic, but which I prefer calling the 'foundations' of bronchoscopic practice. This includes technical skills, and everything linked to the multidisciplinary and multidimensional patient care environment in which informed patients participate actively in management decisions.

Traditionally, numbers of procedures were a metric upon which attaining competency was based. However, a purely numbers-based training program does not equate to competency, and is insufficient on its own[2,3]. Numbers represent hands-on experience in the patient-care setting, but without oversight and structured feedback by trained teachers/mentors, they are of little value. Oversight might take the form of direct observation, distance-monitoring in real-time, or post-hoc reviews of recorded case videos. Feedback through two-way instructor-learner communication based on the use of objective measures or checklists will help improve knowledge and technical skills for both observed as well as hypothetical procedure-related issues.

We believe, therefore, that every hospital department should provide bronchoscopists with manikins or affordable and ideally, free access to simulation so they and their teams can maintain and improve their skills through repetitive, task-driven practice[4,5]. I am constantly puzzled as to why so many university hospitals around the world still refuse to commit small amounts of money to purchase such models so their faculty and trainees might improve and maintain their skills without causing undue suffering or prolonged procedures in patients.

Of course, there is still debate regarding how assessment tools might serve as measures of competency. Score-based assessments if conducted serially, can identify weaknesses to be remedied by individualized training, thus establishing a minimum standard of competency that is potentially confirmed using a high-stakes examination with cut-off scores or pass/fail criteria. This approach helps assure patient safety as well as the ethical and appropriate performance of a particular procedure often required by hospital accreditation committees in credentialing individual practitioners. Other assessments might include multiple-choice style examinations to document learner participation in a predefined number of workshops, charting observations of a learner's behavior during interactive small-group exercises, mandating completion of a specified duration of apprentice-style training, and reviewing procedure-related experience with videos and procedural logbooks.[6,7,8]

Given the above, we caution against learning by doing. Instead, we suggest learners participate in structured, multidimensional educational programs, albeit with a caveat: All learners have varying levels of experience. Some are already competent proceduralists whilst others are beginners, and of course, one may even be an expert in one procedure, yet have novice or intermediate abilities in another. Allowing for individualization and acknowledging that all learners learn differently, adds value to a learner-centric educational approach. Furthermore, training programs should nurture ethical behaviors and scientific curiosity through active participation and growing responsibilities in multidisciplinary interdepartmental meetings, research projects, teaching of more junior colleagues, and by giving an increased place to arguably "soft medicine" subjects alongside science and technology at national conferences and workshops. The role of mentoring is undeniable, and even decision-making and communication skills can be learned. The purpose of our Train-the Trainers programs has been to help teach teachers how to teach. Bronchoscopy

International has conducted more than forty such programs all over the world, and they are received with great enthusiasm, resulting also in a number of certified and master instructors who are able to carry on the mission in their own countries and regions.

We believe that dedicated teaching moments are preferable to teaching on-the-job during clinical/service rounds because most learners have facts, figures, and much of the published literature at their fingertips using mobile devices. In regards to structured curricula and implementing a more uniform model for IP education, the United States now has several 12 to 24-month programs with centralized application processes, published standards for program curricula, and exit examinations. Italy has an extensive curriculum for IP training, including a Master's program through the University of Florence, and, more recently Ancona, providing a link between an academic university-based program for didactic and course-oriented studies with affiliated teaching hospitals to provide the necessary hands-on procedural experience. The European Respiratory Society has an IP accreditation program built around EBUS, and a professional certification program covering theory, online self-directed modules, quizzes, webcasts, course and live case attendance, hands-on simulation training, and submission of a logbook and video cases for review, The Thoracic Society of Australia and New Zealand instituted regional training seminars, procedural log reviews, and encourages using a variety of validated assessment tools while actively building a cadre of Bronchoscopy International® certified and master instructors. In Argentina, a one-year certification program in bronchoscopy includes a multidimensional curriculum, objective measures of knowledge and technical skill, procedural log reviews, multiple opportunities for targeted practice using airway models and manikins, and supervised hands-on training. Similar programs are being designed elsewhere in South America, Romania, Serbia, India, Bangladesh, Malaysia, Indonesia, and Algeria.[9,10,11,12,13]

Technical skills require *muscle memory*. Research shows that neural pathways can be formed, and habits developed by combining many small tasks learned incrementally before combining them into more complex procedures. These skills can be practiced and perfected using inanimate models and computer-based simulation[14,15]. This is similar to the way one learns to play a musical instrument or swing a golf club. We believe that training programs that allow individualization through the identification of strengths and weaknesses using such objective measures also help identify a minimum standard of competency that might be universally accepted regardless of one's country or region of practice. The "Step by Step" method of bronchoscopy training is one example of gradual acquisition of muscle memory whereby trainees acquire skills by deconstructing a complex procedure into numbered steps that are taught individually and combined gradually until the entire procedure is performed[16].

In a multidimensional, structured learning environment, the acquisition of psychomotor skills is ideally accompanied by the acquisition of cognitive (theoretical, metacognitive, and factual), affective (growth in how feelings and emotions might affect decision-making), and experiential (as opposed to a-priori) knowledge. This is accomplished through minor alterations to the apprenticeship-style model and lends credence to the use of small group, case-based instruction using real or fabricated case scenarios. We have incorporated role-playing exercises into our Train-the-Trainer programs with great success and participation satisfaction. Role-playing exercises are also beneficial and popular for practicing communication skills. Independent learning in our programs is encouraged using social media platforms and programs designed for mobile devices. Online resources include Bronchoscopy International® (www.Bronchoscopy.org); Uptodate® in Pulmonary Medicine; Panminerva Medica's comprehensive articles on training needs, competency requirements, and state-of-the-art reviews; online bronchoscopy simulation and YouTube instructional videos, Facebook such as www.facebook.com/groups/pleural.hub/; and dozens of national Bronchology groups representing more than 5000 physicians communicating in real-time using WhatsApp. This forum was of incredible value during the recent SARS-CoV-2 pandemic.

Because time with an instructor is precious, a Flipped Classroom model is also attractive[17]. This differs from a traditional classroom model because materials are usually provided before on-site learning, and students are asked to consider, reflect, and explore content often as homework or during interactive small group sessions. The teacher's role changes from classroom-based lecturer to attentive coach and supportive facilitator. Such an approach lends itself well to problem-based learning methods such as those used in our 4-Box Practical Approach exercises[18].

Hospital-based teaching is usually not done in a formal setting, and frequently, face to face contact between student and teacher occurs at the patient's bedside, in clinical consultation rooms, or the procedure suite. These moments provide priceless opportunities to impart and reinforce knowledge, involve the trainee in care discussions and management plans, provide career advice, and identify a learner's needs. We suggest adding a dedicated moment for teaching, rather than teaching on-the-run, to help distinguish between clinical service (doing the work, providing patient care) and education (where teachers and learners work together to enhance each other's knowledge, skill, and experience).

In regards to using simulation for bronchoscopy training, the existence of commercially available airway manikins and newer disposable bronchoscopes provides a relatively low-cost alternative whilst maintaining a remarkable degree of anatomical realism with a true to life sense of bronchoscope handling. Manikins are often preferable to computer-based simulation for learning to remove foreign bodies, sample endobronchial masses, and suction airway secretions or blood. A single-use disposable bronchoscope costing a few hundred dollars can be reserved for educational purposes and used hundreds of times coupled with an inexpensive display panel[19,20]. A 3D printed airway cast, being a less expensive, custom-made device, may provide even more realism than many expensive commercial units[21].

Results from simulation studies show a demonstrable increase in the acquisition of dexterity skills, improvements in the speed of airway inspection, numbers of segments visualized, reduced airway wall collisions and faster performance on the learning curve early in training; as few as 20 simulated procedures is significantly associated with increased acquisition of bronchoscopy skills on validated assessment tasks. Studies also show superior performance in patients for trainees who learned initially on a simulator compared to those who did not, a finding that is consistent with results from simulator studies in other subspecialties. Laptop-sized models are also available and can be carried to courses.[22,23,24,25,26,27]

If competency is defined as a combination of observable and measurable skills, knowledge, and behaviors, it follows that an assessment strategy using a collection of specific tools and methodologies is required. Among others, these encompass objective forms for measuring, monitoring, and reviewing one's technical skill and knowledge, as well as one's ability to plan a procedure, obtain results similar to those of one's peers, and respond appropriately to procedure-related complications. As alluded to earlier, we also believe competency should be demonstrated in peri-procedural aspects of care such as the ability to obtain informed consent, deliver news of a diagnosis in a culturally sensitive and appropriate manner, communicate effectively with colleagues and patients, perform effectively as a team leader, and develop a satisfactory follow-up procedural plan. This should be accompanied with a greater knowledge and understanding of how medical ethics are applied to interventional pulmonology.

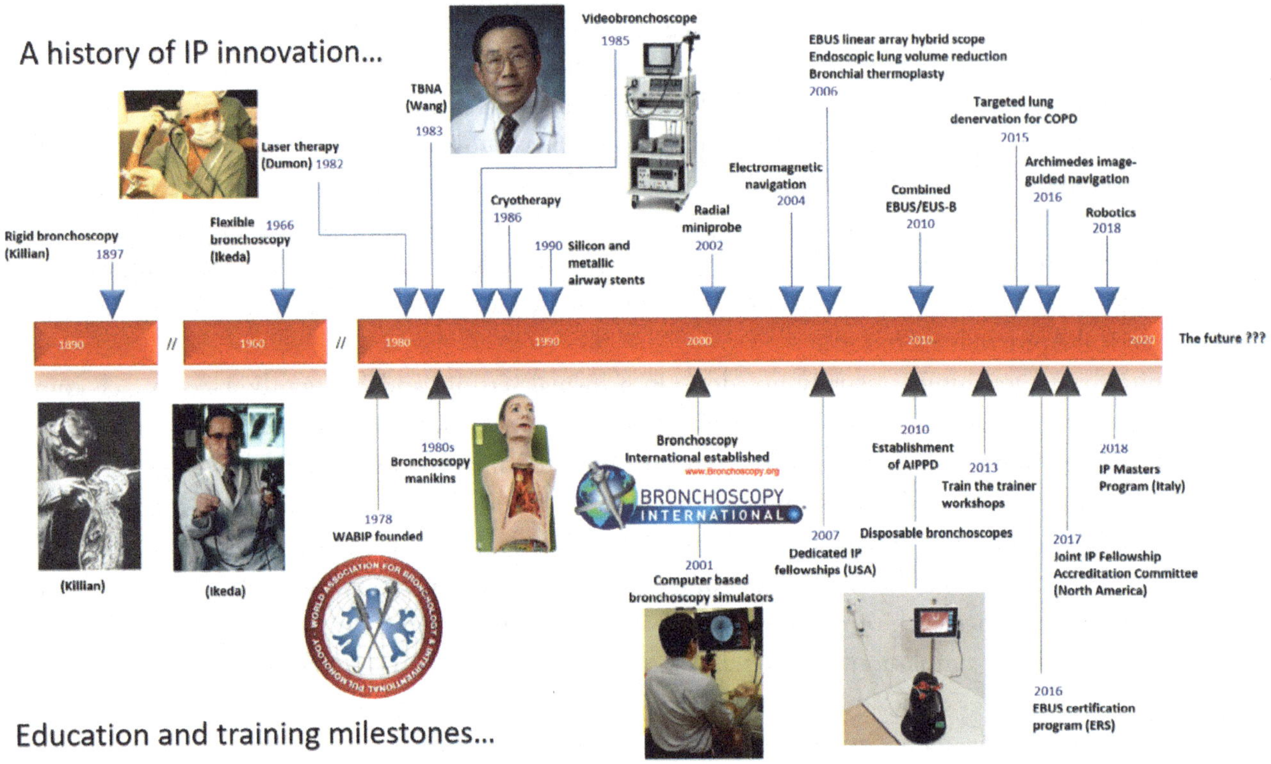

History of IP Innovation. From Colt HG, Williamson JP. Training in interventional pulmonology: What we have learned and a way forward. Respirology. 2020 Sep;25(9):997-1007

References

1. Colleges AoAM. 2018 Fall applicant and matriculant data tables. Association of American Medical Colleges; 2018 December 2018.
2. Wahidi MM, Silvestri G, Conforti J, et al. Assessment of pulmonary fellow acquisition of bronchoscopy skills. *Chest*. 2007;132(4):514C.
3. Downie G, Bowling M, Silvestri G, et al. The Multi-State Bronchoscopy Education Project: acquisition of cognitive skills. *Chest Journal*. 2007;132.
4. Voduc N, Dudek N, Parker CM, et al. Development and Validation of a Bronchoscopy Competence Assessment Tool in a Clinical Setting. *Ann Am Thorac Soc*. 2016;13(4):495-501.
5. Wahidi MM, Silvestri GA, Coakley RD, et al. A prospective multicenter study of competency metrics and educational interventions in the learning of bronchoscopy among new pulmonary fellows. *Chest*. 2010;137(5):1040-9.
6. Salamonsen MR, Bashirzadeh F, Ritchie AJ, et al. A new instrument to assess physician skill at chest tube insertion: the TUBE-iCOMPT. *Thorax*. 2015;70(2):186-8.
7. Dalal PG, Dalal GB, Pott L, et al. Learning curves of novice anesthesiology residents performing simulated fibreoptic upper airway endoscopy. *Can J Anaesth*. 2011;58(9):802-9.
8. Corbetta L, Arru LB, Mereu C, et al. Competence and training in interventional pulmonology. *Panminerva Med*. 2019;61(3):203-31.
9. Mullon JJ, Burkart KM, Silvestri G, et al. Interventional Pulmonology Fellowship Accreditation Standards: Executive Summary of the Multisociety Interventional Pulmonology Fellowship Accreditation Committee. *Chest*. 2017;151(5):1114-21.

10. Corbetta L, Patelli M. Executive Summary of Training and Competence Standards for the Interventional Pulmonology Master Program in Italy. *J Bronchology Interv Pulmonol.* 2018;25(1):6-8.
11. Williamson JP, Twaddell SH, Lee YCG, et al. Thoracic ultrasound recognition of competence: A position paper of the Thoracic Society of Australia and New Zealand. *Respirology.* 2017;22(2):405-8.
12. Miller GE. The assessment of clinical skills/competence/performance. *Acad Med.* 1990;65(9 Suppl):S63-7.
13. Farr A, Clementsen P, Herth F, et al Endobronchial ultrasound: launch of an ERS structured training programme. *Breathe.* 2016;12(3):217-20.
14. Davoudi M, Osann K, Colt HG. Validation of two instruments to assess technical bronchoscopic skill using virtual reality simulation. *Respiration.* 2008;76(1):92-101.
15. Ost D, Rosiers AD, Britt EJ, et ale. Assessment of a Bronchoscopy Simulator. *American Journal of Respiratory and Critical Care Medicine.* 2001;164(12):2248-55.
16. 54. Bronchoscopy International [cited 2019 7-12-2019]. Available from: https://bronchoscopy.org/step-by-step.
17. Baker JW. The "Classroom Flip": Using Web course management tools to become the guide by the side. In: Chambers JA, editor. Selected papers from the 11th International Conference on College Teaching and Learning. Jacksonville, Florida: Florida Community College at Jacksonville; 2000. p. 9-17.
18. Colt HG and Murgu S. *Bronchoscopy and Central Airways Obstruction*: A Patient-Centered Approach. New York, Saunders 2012.
19. Baker PA, Weller JM, Baker MJ, et al. Evaluating the ORSIM(R) simulator for assessment of anaesthetists' skills in flexible bronchoscopy: aspects of validity and reliability. *Br J Anaesth.* 2016;117 Suppl 1:i87-i91.
20. Garner JL, Garner SD, Hardie RJ, et al. Evaluation of a re-useable bronchoscopy biosimulator with ventilated lungs. *ERJ Open Res.* 2019;5(2):00035-2019.
21. Pedersen TH, Gysin J, Wegmann A, et al. A randomised, controlled trial evaluating a low cost, 3D-printed bronchoscopy simulator. *Anaesthesia.* 2017;72(8):1005-9.
22. Blum MG, Powers TW, Sundaresan S. Bronchoscopy simulator effectively prepares junior residents to competently perform basic clinical bronchoscopy. *Ann Thorac Surg.* 2004;78(1):287-91; discussion -91.
23. Cook DA, Hatala R, Brydges R, et al. Technology-enhanced simulation for health professions education: a systematic review and meta-analysis. *Jama.* 2011;306(9):978-88.
24. Clay AS, Gold JA. Teaching with Simulation. In: Kritek PA, Richards JB, editors. Medical Education in Pulmonary, Critical Care, and Sleep Medicine: Advanced Concepts and Strategies. Cham: Springer International Publishing; 2019. p. 213-33.
25. Konge L, Arendrup H, von Buchwald C, et al. Using Performance in Multiple Simulated Scenarios to Assess Bronchoscopy Skills. *Respiration.* 2011;81(6):483-90.
26. Colt HG, Davoudi M, Murgu S, et al. Measuring learning gain during a one-day introductory bronchoscopy course. *Surg Endosc.* 2011;25(1):207-16.
27. Miller RJ, Mudambi L, Vial MR, et al. Evaluation of Appropriate Mediastinal Staging among Endobronchial Ultrasound Bronchoscopists. *Ann Am Thorac Soc.* 2017;14(7):1162-8.

****

Endobronchial Ultrasound and EBUS-TBNA Program Learning Objectives

This program is designed for long-term use. Learners will acquire and improve on their skills during a lifetime of learning and practice. Practitioners may wish to enter this program in order to improve or supplement their knowledge and skills. Others will participate in this program as part of their subspecialty training.

The program was developed so that parts could be learned by participating in regional seminars. Other aspects of the program will require dedicated study and practice during the course of one's training.

By the end of this program, participants will have achieved the following objectives:

- Acquired cognitive knowledge of endobronchial ultrasound and bronchoscopic practice as demonstrated by passing scores on the Essential EBUS Bronchoscopist©.
- Acquired technical skill enabling the independent performance of EBUS and EBUS-Guided TBNA by demonstrating passing scores on EBUS step-by-step, EBUS-STAT, and proctored checklists.
- Acquired cognitive, technical, affective, and experiential knowledge and skills as required in case of consultation for convex probe EBUS bronchoscopy as documented by passing scores on the patient-centered practical approach exercise checklist.
- Ability to describe and perform the major elements of informed consent, moderate sedation, procedural pause, and patient safety (image processor and safety) as demonstrated by 100% passing scores on each of the associated checklists.
- Ability to technically perform endobronchial ultrasound and EBUS-Guided TBNA, use common nomenclature, and recognize imaging patters as documented by passing scores using EBUS-BSTAT and on-line independent study of images and instructional videos such as those included in BronchAtlas™.
- Acquired confidence performing EBUS and EBUS-TBNA as documented using EBUS-SAT.

Endobronchial Ultrasound and EBUS-GUIDED TBNA Curriculum contains:

1. *Endobronchial Ultrasound and EBUS-TBNA Competency Program Completion Checklist*
2. *Regional EBUS and EBUS-TBNA courses* comprised of didactic lectures, interactive sessions and simulation-based hands-on workshops using a pre-test/post-test model to document cognitive knowledge and technical skill acquisition.
3. Reading assignments:
    - *The EBUS Bronchoscopist©*, a single module, 30 question/answer Web-based study guide with downloadable PDF files and 10 question post-test (mandatory).
    - *Lung Cancer Staging (Revised IASLC)* and *EBUS Lymph Node Map* Module with didactic lecture, synopsis and video (optional).
    - *EBUS-CT-White Light Bronchoscopy Correlations* Module with didactic lecture, synopsis (poster) and video (optional).
    - *Ultrasound Physics and Terminology* Module with didactic lecture, synopsis, and video (optional).
    - *Tumor Markers and Clinical Pathway exercise*
    - *Moderate Sedation* Module with lecture, synopsis and associated checklist.
4. The *EBUS Step-by-Step* procedural skill acquisition
5. A series of *simulation workshops* that include:
    - An *EBUS Informed Consent*, *EBUS Patient Safety*, and *EBUS Procedural Pause* simulation.
    - An *EBUS Airway Access and Image Acquisition* simulation including introduction of the EBUS bronchoscope through a laryngeal mask airway, endotracheal tube, and oral bite block. Uses inanimate models in order to demonstrate the use of color Doppler, gain, depth, frequency and focus adjustments.
    - An *EBUS-TBNA needle and scope handling* simulation using inanimate models and/or high-fidelity computer-based simulation to sample lymph node stations.
6. A series of *observed real-patient encounters* which include:
    - An *EBUS airway access and image acquisition* encounter (using the EBUS processor needle and scope handling checklist).
    - A patient encounter warranting review of informed consent, procedural pause, universal precautions and related checklists.
    - An *EBUS-TBNA* encounter (using EBUS-STAT).

7. A series of interactive (instructor-student) *Patient-centered practical approach to procedural decision-making* workshops.
8. A *proctored real patient (CP) EBUS-TBNA bronchoscopy* with competency assessment.
9. A collection of *assessment* tools used to monitor progress:
    - Endobronchial Skills and Tasks Assessment Tool (EBUS-STAT)
    - Endobronchial Ultrasound Self-Assessment Tool (EBUS-SAT)
10. A collection of *Checklists* used to monitor progress and help assure patient safety:
    - EBUS Informed Consent checklist
    - EBUS Sedation-Anesthesia checklist
    - EBUS Procedural Pause checklist
    - EBUS Processor and needle checklist
    - EBUS Practical Approach checklist
    - EBUS Proctored EBUS-TBNA checklist

****

SECTION 1

Regional Courses

Regional programs are comprised of didactic lectures, interactive sessions and simulation-based hands-on workshops, often using a pre-test/post-test model to document cognitive knowledge and technical skill acquisition.

USER INSTRUCTIONS

Regional Courses (1 day) EBUS and EBUS-TBNA

Learning bronchoscopy in the clinical setting promotes learner anxiety, forces patients to suffer the burden of medical procedure-related learning [1], and results in a highly variable learning experience [2]. Clinical responsibilities often interfere with reading of bronchoscopy-related material, and, in the absence of periodic assessments of bronchoscopy-related knowledge, trainees are unlikely to be compliant with educational endeavors they perceive as optional or reliant on individual motivation, especially if there are no pass/fail grading consequences [3]. The current subspecialty bronchoscopy learning environment is further rendered less-than-ideal for beginners because of concerns regarding patient safety, fiscal constraints, and an increasing impetus to document procedural competency [4-6].

Whilst not supplanting on-the-job training that occurs with subspecialty rotations, short postgraduate courses comprised of lectures and simulation-based hands-on instruction, have thus become a popular means towards enhancing procedure-related learning [7-9]. In accordance with continued medical education (CME) guidelines, these programs identify learner objectives and provide opportunities for feedback from students regarding the perceived quality of the course.

The purpose of regional courses is to provide standardized learning material to bronchoscopy trainees. By regionalizing the process, program directors can enlist participants from numerous regional programs, thereby reducing course-related expenditures pertaining to travel and lodging. Already, several courses have become highly popular in the Carolinas, Southern California, and Midwest. Other regional courses are occurring in the Asia, Latin America and Australia. During course participation, learners are exposed to uniform course material delivered using didactic lectures, interactive sessions, hands-on training using patient models, low-fidelity and high-fidelity simulation, debriefing exercises, and problem-based learning modules. Pre-test/post-test assessments help document knowledge and technical skill acquisition, thereby setting a new baseline for learners in subspecialty training.

It has long been recognized that assessment drives learning, and that rigorous assessment inspires learning, reinforces confidence, and reassures the public. Proving that course participation is responsible for learning gains is difficult. For example, demonstrating the short-term benefit of an educational intervention is controversial because of debates regarding the value of pre-test and post-test assessments, and because of the obvious difficulty constituting a control group to which studies of an educational intervention can be compared [10-13]. Studies of long-term retention are problematic because causality is subject to the effects of normal maturation and ongoing training history [14].

The true value of pre-test/post-test assessments has also been controversial because of the effects of many extraneous variables, which include the Hawthorne effect (knowing that one is being tested may affect the results), the halo effect (the human tendency to respond positively or negatively to an instructor), and the practice effect (of a pre-test on a subsequent post-test). In the context of procedure-based training, the calculation of various measures of learning gain, including class-average and single-student normalized gain provides an objective and informative means to document learner performance and demonstrate robustness of the educational intervention.

Patients should not suffer the burden of procedure-related learning. Participation in regional courses, using simulation-based deliberate practice to acquire technical skill, and documenting a rapid climb up the initially steep slope of the novice's learning curve should result in decreased patient suffering and improved procedure-related decision making. Diverse opinions regarding educational methodologies, curricular structure, and measures of effectiveness persist in regards to short one- or two-day programs [15-16]. Additional studies are needed to document effectiveness and to determine how regional courses might favorably impact patient outcomes.

Selected References

1. Silvestri GA. The evolution of bronchoscopy training. Respiration. 2008;76(1):92-101.
2. Haponik EF, Russell GB, Beamis JF, et al. Bronchoscopy training: current fellows' experiences and some concerns for the future. Chest. 2000 Sep;118(3):572-573.
3. Wahidi MM, Silvestri GA, Coakley RD, Ferguson JS, Shepherd RW, Moses L, Conforti J, Que L, Anstrom KJ, McGuire F, Colt H, Downie GH. A prospective multi-center study of competency metrics and educational interventions in the learning of bronchoscopy among starting pulmonary fellows. Chest 2010;137(5):1040-1049.
4. Reznick RK, MacRae H. Teaching Surgical Skills – Changes in the Wind. N Engl J Ned. 2006; 355:2664-2669.
5. Carraccio C, Englander R. Evaluating competence using a portfolio: a literature review and web-based application to the ACGME competencies. Teach Learn Med. 2004 Fall;16(4):381-387.
6. Carraccio C, Wolfsthal SD, Englander R, et al. Shifting Paradigms: From Flexner to Competencies. Academic Medicine. 2002;77(5):361-367.
7. Norman G. The American College of Chest Physicians evidence-based educational guidelines for continuing medical education interventions: a critical review of evidence-based educational guidelines. Chest. 2009;135(3):834-837.
8. Schijven MP, Schout BM, Dolmans VE, Hendrikx AJ, Broeders IA, Borel Rinkes IH. Perceptions of surgical specialists in general surgery, orthopaedic surgery, urology and gynaecology on teaching endoscopic surgery in The Netherlands. Surg Endosc. 2008;22(2):472-482.
9. Davis D, Bordage G, Moores LK, Bennett N, Marinopoulos SS, Mazmanian PE, Dorman T, McCrory D. The Science of Continuing Medical Education. Chest.2009;135:8S-16S.
10. Cronbach LJ, Furby L. How should we measure "change" or should we? Psychol. Bull 1970;74:68-80.
11. Hake, R.R. 2009. "Should We Measure Change? Yes!" <http://www.physics.indiana.edu/~hake>. And <http://www.physics.indiana.edu/~hake/MeasChangeS.pdf> (2.5 MB)
12. Melzer DE. Normalized learning gain: A key measure of student learning [Addendum to: Melzer DE. The relationship between mathematics preparation and conceptual learning gains in physics: A possible "hidden variable" in diagnostic pretest scores. Am J. Phys 2002;70:1259-1267. Online http://scitation.aip.org/getpdf/servlet/GetPDFServlet?filetype=pdf&id=AJPIAS000070000012001259000001&idtype=cvips [Accessed June 16, 2009].
13. USDE. 2003. U.S. Department of Education, Identifying and Implementing Educational Practices Supported by Rigorous Evidence: A User Friendly Guide. Institute of Education Sciences, National Center for Education

Evaluation and Regional Assistance. The entire guide is online at <http://www.ed.gov/rschstat/research/pubs/rigorousevid/index.html> / "PDF (140KB)".

14. Shadish, W.R., T.D. Cook, & D.T. Campbell. 2002. Experimental and Quasi-Experimental Designs for Generalized Causal Inference. Houghton Mifflin - information at <http://tinyurl.com/y3e7vw>.
15. Colt HG, Davoudi M, Murgu SD, Zamanian Rohani N. Colt HG, Davoudi M, Murgu S, and Rohani NZ. Measuring learning gain during a one-day introductory bronchoscopy course. Surgical Endoscopy 2010;25:207-216.
16. Colt HG, Davoudi M, Quadrelli S, Rohani N. Competency-based metrics to measure short-term knowledge and skill acquisition during a two-day thoracoscopy program. Respiration 2010;80(6):553-559.

Endobronchial Ultrasound and EBUS-TBNA

One day program with didactic lectures, interactive sessions, and hands-on workshops. Example of program objectives and methods.

Program Objectives

At the end of this one-day program that includes didactic, interactive, and hands-on training sessions, the program participant will have:

- Increased factual knowledge of endobronchial ultrasound including aspects of:
  - Patient safety, equipment safety, prevention and response to complications
  - Expected results and greater knowledge of mediastinal anatomy
  - Lung cancer staging, tumor markers and specimen handling
  - Techniques, CT-Bronchoscopy-EBUS correlations and pattern recognition
- Enhanced medical decision-making ability
- Improved technical skill performing endobronchial ultrasound and convex probe EBUS-guided transbronchial needle aspiration.

Methods used to accomplish program objectives

- Didactic lectures
- Interactive sessions
- Patient-centered problem-based learning exercises
- Hands-on technical skill training using lo-fidelity inanimate airway models and hi-fidelity simulation.
- Instructor-led small group interactive exercises pertaining to equipment handling, informed consent and patient safety, mediastinal anatomy, and pattern recognition.
- Assessment of technical skill performing endobronchial ultrasound using validated bronchoscopy assessment tools (EBUS-SAT and EBUS-STAT) if time allows.
- Post course written knowledge assessment with general review of correct answers.

Example of a One-day EBUS & EBUS-TBNA Program

7:30-8:15 am	Registration, pre-test and survey of practice experience
8:15-8:30	Welcome, introduction, and learning objectives
8:30-9:00	EBUS-TBNA Indications, diagnostic yield, complications
9:00-9:30	EBUS-TBNA Technique and smear preparation
9:30-10:00	Mediastinal anatomy (IASLC) and lymph node structure
10:00-10:15	EBUS-CT-White light bronchoscopy correlations
10:15-10:30	BREAK
10:30-11:00	EBUS: Other applications
11:00-11:30	Practical Approach to EBUS-TBNA
11:30-12:00	Interactive session: EBUS-TBNA True/False exercises
12:00-1:00	LUNCH
Afternoon hands-on training 1:00-3:30 pm	Hands-on training: 4 stations – minimum 35 minutes per station (1) EBUS Step by Step: handling the scope and the needle (x2) (2) EBUS Step by Step: handling the scope and the image (x2) (3) Nodal and vascular mediastinal anatomy: pattern recognition (4) Patient-based Practical Approach to EBUS-TBNA
3:30-4:15	Post course technical skills and cognitive learning assessments
4:15-4:30	Wrap up, certificate of course completion

EBUS and EBUS-TBNA: Hands-On Workstations

Workstation 1: EBUS Step by Step: Scope and Needle Handling

Learning Objectives:

1. To be able to demonstrate how to move the EBUS scope into position.
2. To be able to demonstrate techniques of needle insertion and EBUS-TBNA.
3. To demonstrate communication skills with bronchoscopy assistants.

Description:

The instructor will review the *EBUS-TBNA Step by Step Instructional Video* with the group. EBUS-TBNA will be performed through the carina into subcarinal adenopathy of the specially designed lo-fidelity EBUS airway model, followed by EBUS-TBNA at levels 7, 4R and 4l. The instructor will describe different ways with which to assure patient and operator safely, and ways in which the EBUS bronchoscope is protected. Each team member will demonstrate needle insertion techniques, while another team member serves as the bronchoscopy assistant, assuring patient, operator, and equipment safety. This instructional session focuses on repetition and focused practice.

Workstation 2: EBUS Step by Step: Scope and Image Handling

Learning Objectives:

1. To be able to turn on and set up the EBUS processor
2. To be able to introduce the EBUS scope using Laryngeal mask intubation (LMA), endotracheal intubation, or the bronchoscopic transoral route.
3. To be able to manipulate the scope atraumatically inside the artificial airway and inside the upper and lower airways.
4. To demonstrate the use of gain, and depth and Doppler for image acquisition.
5. To be able to trouble-shoot complications and equipment malfunction.

Description:

The instructor will review the *EBUS Physics Instructional Video* with the group. Students will be asked to make changes on the image processor in order to better visualize the target lymph node at levels 7, 4R or RL using the specially-designed lo-fidelity model. Intubation in the patient with an EBUS scope can be difficult. Because EBUS can be performed using different intubation techniques, the operator will demonstrate the ability to manipulate the scope in the artificial airway prior to obtaining an EBUS image.

Workstation 3: Nodal and vascular mediastinal anatomy: pattern recognition

Learning Objectives:

1. To be able to precisely elaborate a strategy for nodal sampling using computed tomography scans for planning an EBUS-TBNA procedure.
2. To be able to recognize site-specific EBUS imaging of mediastinal and hilar nodal and vascular anatomy.

Description:

The instructor will review the *EBUS Lymph node map Instructional Video* with the group. The instructor will demonstrate how a CT scan can be used to plan an EBUS-TBNA procedure, after which team members will be asked to elaborate a procedural strategy based on an imaging study. During this small group, interactive session, participants will then study a collection of site-specific images corresponding to nodal and vascular, mediastinal and hilar anatomy.

Workstation 4: Patient-based Practical Approach to EBUS-TBNA

Learning Objectives:

1. The learner should be able to identify case-specific elements that are important for procedural strategy and planning.
2. The learner should be able to describe technical elements critical for the execution of EBUS-TBNA, including review of CT scan and choosing nodal sampling strategies.
3. The learner should be able to identify procedure-related risks, benefits, and alternatives, as well as have a plan of action in case of procedure-related complications.

Description:

In this interactive session, the instructor opens the floor to the learners, and together they walk through a patient's clinical scenario using the 4-Box Practical Approach model, working their way through initial patient evaluation, assessment of procedural strategies (including indications and contraindications, expected results, and risk-benefit analysis), discuss procedural techniques and results (including choosing among technical options and instruments, knowing the anatomic risks, results, and possible complications and how to deal with each), and devising long-term management plans (including assessment of the results, plan for follow-up diagnostic and therapeutic options, along with quality improvement for the procedural team). This "Practical Approach" exercise combines cognitive, theoretical technical, affective, and experiential learning.

§

Example of a One-day EBUS Program using mostly interactive sessions

7:30-8:00 am	Registration, Coffee and Continental breakfast
8:00-8:15	Introduction and Learning objectives
8:15-8:30	EBUS Bronchoscopist: interactive Q& A
8:30-9:00	Lymph Node Sampling and Specimen Processing
9:00-9:15	EBUS Bronchoscopist: interactive Q& A
9:15-9:45	Surgical Mediastinal Staging (IASLC)
9:45-10:00	EBUS Bronchoscopist: interactive Q& A
10:00-10:15	BREAK
10:15-11:45	Station 1: CT- Bronchoscopy – EBUS correlations: interactive session
10:15-11:45	Station 2: EBUS Mediastinal Lymph Node Mapping: interactive video session
10:15-11:45	Station 3: Specimen handling and Smear preparation: hands on session
11:45-12:45	LUNCH
12:45-13:15	EBUS Applied Physics
13:15-13:30	EBUS Bronchoscopist: interactive Q& A
13:30-14:00	Results and Complications of EBUS-TBNA
14:00-14:30	EBUS-TBNA: multimodal imaging guidance and molecular analysis for EBUS-TBNA
14:30-14:45	BREAK
14:45-16:15	Station 4: EBUS technique step by step: hands on session
14:45-16:15	Station 5: EBUS technique step by step: hands on session
14:45-16:15	Station 6: EBUS technique step by step: hands on session
16:15-16:30	Certificate of attendance ceremony, acknowledgement of guest faculty
16:30-17:00	Tea time

Equipment Needs:

- EBUS stations and all EBUS accessories/needles (Stations 4,5,6)
- Lo-fidelity EBUS models (stations 4,5,6)
- Color handouts of EBUS-STAT (Stations 4,5, 6) with clipboards
- Laptop computers and large screen computer display panels (Stations 1, 2)
- Interactive audience participation software (EBUS bronchoscopist Q&A)
- EBUS needles, syringes and specimen preparation accessories (tubes, solutions, slides) for stains, cultures and flow cytometry (Station 3)
- Attendee's package: UCI clipboard with notepad; EBUS-STAT handout; schedule; name tag; EBUS-CT-WLB poster; certificate and USB drive with videos, lectures as PDF files and EBUS bronchoscopist PDF file

Workstation objectives

Station 1: CT-Bronchoscopy-EBUS correlations Learning Objectives:

1. To understand the correlations between computed tomography scanning planes and EBUS images for mediastinal and hilar lymph nodes based on revised IASLC system.
2. To be able to integrate CT with bronchoscopic findings for planning EBUS-TBNA.

Description: The instructor will first demonstrate the step-by-step principles for correlating the CT images with the EBUS images displayed on the monitor. It is important for each learner to become fully aware of the reference points used for this process, the EBUS transducer scanning plane and the CT planes. Using flash cards, during this interactive session, the learners will be asked to match a CT image of a particular lymph node station with its corresponding EBUS image.

Station 2: EBUS Lymph Node Mapping Learning Objectives:

1. To be able to demonstrate the correct position and orientation of the EBUS transducer in the airway for visualizing a particular lymph node station
2. To be able to describe the surrounding structures for a particular hilar or mediastinal lymph node on EBUS display

Description: The instructor will first demonstrate the step-by-step principles and techniques for hilar and mediastinal lymph node mapping on EBUS. Each learner will then be required to describe and demonstrate the visualization of a specific lymph node station and review the mediastinal anatomy using the high-fidelity simulator and flash cards.

Station 3: Specimen Handling and Smear Preparation Learning Objectives:

1. To be able to demonstrate correct specimen placement on the slides and tubing
2. To be able to demonstrate two correct slide preparation techniques
3. To be able to describe the specific specimen assignment for cell block, flow cytometry, immuno-histochemistry and mutation analysis

Description: The instructor and the assistant will first demonstrate step by step principles and techniques for specimen handling, slide preparation and processing. It is important for each learner to become fully aware of the type of specimens obtained (slides, cell block, tissue core), their proper handling and processing for diagnosis and downstream molecular analysis. During this session, each student will also learn the specific specimen processing for a particular molecular marker used in personalized cancer treatment.

Station 4: EBUS technique step by step Learning Objectives:

1. To be able to turn on and set up the EBUS processor
2. To demonstrate the use of Doppler, gain, and depth
3. To be able to trouble-shoot complications and equipment malfunction.
4. To be able to demonstrate use of the EBUS needle.

Description: The instructor will first demonstrate step by step principles and techniques for using the processor and needle. It will be essential for each learner to become fully aware of equipment functions and malfunctions, as well as with the functioning of the EBUS-needle.

Station 5: EBUS technique step by step Learning Objectives:

1. To be able to demonstrate techniques of needle insertion and EBUS-TBNA.
2. To be able to demonstrate communication skills with nursing assistants.
3. To be able to demonstrate use of EBUS and white light bronchoscopy
4. To be able to identify major lymph node stations.

Description: The instructor will first demonstrate EBUS and EBUS-TBNA with the help of a bronchoscopy assistant. EBUS-TBNA will be performed through the carina into subcarinal adenopathy of the specially lo-fidelity airway model, followed by EBUS-TBNA at the level 4R and 4L regions. The instructor will also describe different ways with which to assure patient and operator safely, and ways in which the EBUS bronchoscope is protected. Each team member will then demonstrate needle insertion techniques, while another team member serves as the bronchoscopy assistant, making sure that patient, operator, and equipment safety is assured.

Station 6: EBUS technique step by step Learning Objectives:

1. To be able to demonstrate techniques of needle insertion and EBUS-TBNA.
2. To be able to demonstrate communication skills with nursing assistants.

3. To be able to demonstrate use of EBUS and white light bronchoscopy
4. To be able to identify major lymph node stations.

Description: The instructor will first demonstrate EBUS and EBUS-TBNA with the help of a bronchoscopy assistant. EBUS-TBNA will be performed through the carina into subcarinal adenopathy of the specially lo-fidelity airway model, followed by EBUS-TBNA at the level 4R and 4L regions. The instructor will also describe different ways with which to assure patient and operator safely, and ways in which the EBUS bronchoscope is protected. Each team member will then demonstrate needle insertion techniques, while another team member serves as the bronchoscopy assistant, making sure that patient, operator, and equipment safety is assured.

Example of EBUS-TBNA Training Course Evaluation Form

A. Please indicate your position: (Circle) Fellow Faculty (If Faculty, proceed to Item C)

B. How well did this activity meet the following learning objectives? (Circle one)

(Scale for B: 1=not at all, 2=slightly, 3=moderately, 4=mostly, 5=completely)

Course Objectives					
Increased my knowledge of lymph node stations, sampling techniques and specimen processing	1	2	3	4	5
Improved my understanding and memory of mediastinal anatomy and lung cancer staging	1	2	3	4	5
Increased my factual knowledge of EBUS pertaining to the use of the processor and instruments	1	2	3	4	5
Increased my knowledge of EBUS-TBNA as it pertains to diagnostic yield and complications	1	2	3	4	5
Increased my knowledge of tumor markers used for personalized therapy	1	2	3	4	5
Increased my ability to integrate CT with bronchoscopic findings for planning EBUS-TBNA	1	2	3	4	5
Improved my technical skill regarding performance of EBUS examination	1	2	3	4	5
Improved my technical skill regarding performance of EBUS-TBNA	1	2	3	4	5

C. **Presentations: Please rate each of the following speaker presentations on their presentation skills, knowledge of content and degree to which presentation was balanced, objective and scientifically rigorous?**

(Scale for C: 1=poor, 2=below average, 3=average, 4=above average, 5=outstanding)

Presentations	Presenter	Presentation Skills	Content, Objectivity & Scientific Rigor
Lymph node sampling and specimen processing	x	1 2 3 4 5	1 2 3 4 5
Surgical Mediastinal Staging (IASLC)	x	1 2 3 4 5	1 2 3 4 5
EBUS Bronchoscopist: interactive Q&A	x	1 2 3 4 5	1 2 3 4 5
EBUS applied physics	x	1 2 3 4 5	1 2 3 4 5
Results and Complications of EBUS-TBNA	x	1 2 3 4 5	1 2 3 4 5
Multimodal imaging guidance and molecular analysis for EBUS-TBNA	x	1 2 3 4 5	1 2 3 4 5

D. **Workshops: Please rate each of the following workshops for the mentor's presentation and the quality of the training models used.**

(Scale for D: 1=poor, 2=below average, 3=average, 4=above average, 5=outstanding)

Workshop	Mentor	Mentor Skills	Fidelity Models
CT-Bronchoscopy-EBUS correlations	x	1 2 3 4 5	1 2 3 4 5
EBUS Mediastinal Lymph Node Mapping	x	1 2 3 4 5	1 2 3 4 5
Specimen handling and smear preparation	x	1 2 3 4 5	1 2 3 4 5
EBUS technique step by step	x	1 2 3 4 5	1 2 3 4 5
EBUS technique step by step	x	1 2 3 4 5	1 2 3 4 5
EBUS technique step by step	x	1 2 3 4 5	1 2 3 4 5

E. **Logistical Items:**

(Scale for E: 1 =poor, 2=below average, 3=average, 4=above average, 5=outstanding)

Logistical Items					
Facilities: Lecture Room	1	2	3	4	5
Facilities: Workshop Rooms	1	2	3	4	5
Food Service	1	2	3	4	5

F. Length of activity: ________ Too short ________ Satisfactory ________ Too long

G. What can be done to improve this educational experience?

____

____

____

____

Thank you for participating in this seminar and for completing this evaluation. We appreciate your input and hope you found the lectures, workshops and time we spent together helpful.

The Bronchoscopy International Team and Guest Faculty

****

SECTION 2

Reading Assignments

1. *The Essential EBUS Bronchoscopist*©: A collection of 30 question/answer sets in the form of a self-study guide and 10 question post-tests.
2. *Lung Cancer Staging* and *EBUS Lymph Node Map:* module with didactic lecture, synopsis, and instructional video.
3. *EBUS-CT-White Light Bronchoscopy Correlations:* module with didactic lecture, synopsis (poster), and instructional video.
4. *EBUS Physics and Terminology:* module with didactic lecture, synopsis, and instructional video.
5. *Moderate Sedation* Module

* Checklists, videos, and post-tests used at the discretion of program director. Videos viewable on You Tube (BronchOrg site) and through www.Bronchoscopy.org.

USER INSTRUCTIONS

Suggested Reading

Suggested reading of the (1) Essential EBUS Bronchoscopist (2) Lung cancer staging (revised IASLC) and EBUS lymph node map module (3) EBUS-CT-White Light bronchoscopy correlations module, and (4) EBUS physics and terminology module, (5) Moderate sedation module

The purpose of these readings is to provide learners with knowledge of basic principles pertaining to Lung cancer staging, EBUS-TBNA mediastinal and hilar lymph node assessments, and EBUS-related ultrasound physics. Reading these assignments will complement reading The Essential EBUS Bronchoscopist. While it is presumed that institutions have their own regulations and protocols, many do not have a formal program of education in these three areas.

Any misunderstandings of general principles in these areas could adversely effect patient management. In addition to reading materials, learners may wish to view specific instructional videos and repeatedly study relevant materials at their own leisure as well as during the course of their training.

We recommend at least ONE formal session during which a didactic lecture on each of these subjects is provided, most beneficial after learners have reviewed the synopsis and other pertinent material such as posters and instructional videos (available on www.Bronchoscopy.org, and the Bronchoscopy International YouTube and Facebook sites).

USER INSTRUCTIONS

The Essential EBUS Bronchoscopist© with post-tests

The *Essential EBUS Bronchoscopist*© is a laddered curriculum of bronchoscopy knowledge prepared after consultation with several EBUS experts worldwide. The text is the second in **The Essential Bronchoscopist® Series**, and is an integral part of the Bronchoscopy Education Project. It is available in Kindle and paperback from Amazon, and downloadable from www.Bronchoscopy.org.

The aim of The *Essential EBUS Bronchoscopist* © is to complement a traditional apprenticeship model of training in EBUS and EBUS-TBNA by emphasizing important facets of knowledge and skill required for competency. Elements addressed in The *Essential EBUS Bronchoscopist* © are intentionally written so that contrary opinions might occasionally be provided by instructors. In this fashion, dialogue is promoted, but access to a certain amount of "essential" material is guaranteed. The question-answer sets of The *Essential EBUS Bronchoscopist*© contain information pertaining to mediastinal and hilar nodal and vascular anatomy, lymph node mapping, scope insertion and placement within the airways, patient preparation, indications, contraindications and complications, techniques and solutions to technical problems, image processing and troubleshooting, ultrasound physics and image artifacts, site specific pattern recognition, as well as lung cancer staging and restaging.

In order to document that a learner has been exposed to material contained in the *Essential EBUS Bronchoscopist*©, a passing score of 70 and above (7/10 correct responses) is recommended to consider the module completed on the EBUS Bronchoscopy Education Competency Checklist.

Selected References

1. Colt HG, Davoudi M, Murgu S. Scientific evidence and principles for use of endobronchial ultrasound and EBUS-TBNA. Expert Rev Med Dev 2011;8(4):493-513.
2. Varela-Lema L, Fernandez-Villar A, Ruano-Ravina A. Effectiveness and safety of endobronchial ultrasound–transbronchial needle aspiration: a systematic review. Eur Respir J 2009; 33: 1156–1164.
3. Nishina K, Hirooka K, Wiegand J, Dremel H. Principles and Practice of endoscopic ultrasound. In Boliger CT et al (eds): Clinical Chest Ultrasound: From the ICU to the bronchoscopy suite. Prog Respir Res. Basel, Karger, 2009;37: 110-127.

4. Steinfort DP, Khor YH, Manser RL, Irving LB. Radial probe endobronchialultrasound for the diagnosis of peripheral lung cancer: systematic review and meta-analysis. Eur Respir J. 2011 Apr;37(4):902-10.
5. Cameron SE, Andrade RS, Pambuccian SE. Endobronchial ultrasound-guided transbronchial needle aspiration cytology: a state-of the art review. Cytopathology. 2010 Feb;21(1):6-26.

Example from The Essential EBUS Bronchoscopist

Question I.3: While performing EBUS-TBNA, you notice that the lymph node being sampled moves but that the needle does not enter it. What should be done next?

A. Abort the procedure
B. Change to a conventional bronchoscope with larger histology needle
C. Change the puncture site
D. Proceed with aspiration anyway

Answer I.3: C

There is usually no reason to abort the procedure or switch to a conventional bronchoscope. Often the needle does not penetrate the node because of the thick capsule of the node, or because the needle is hitting airway cartilage. In the Figure below, images A, B and C were captured at three consecutive moments during EBUS-TBNA. Please notice the LN (the isoechoic oval structure) and its capsule (the hyperechoic line) moving away from the transducer, suggesting that the needle has not penetrated the capsule. In most cases, retracting the needle into the scope, and slightly changing the position of the EBUS scope while still maintaining view of the lymph node, will allow penetration of the node when the needle is advanced again more forcefully, while sometimes minimally changing the position of the needle hub (sheath) on the airway wall. Aspiration should not be performed unless the lymph node is obviously penetrated, as the aspirate will likely reveal benign bronchial cells and be nondiagnostic.

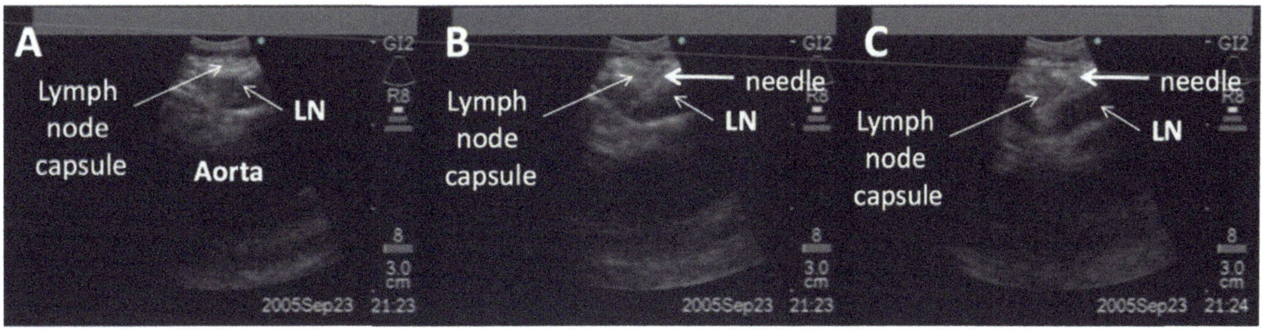

Lung Cancer Staging and EBUS Lymph Nodemap: Synopsis

The purpose of this synopsis is to provide readers with a brief overview of the IASLC Revised Lung Cancer Staging System, particularly effects of stage on prognosis and survival, as well as to provide a description of how EBUS can map mediastinal and hilar nodal and vascular anatomy. It is assumed that institutions and practitioners have different biases and regulations. Herein a summary is provided so that EBUS bronchoscopists might enhance or reinforce their knowledge of nodal staging, lymph node regions, and TNM stage-related prognosis. Readers are encouraged to follow guidelines, protocols and algorithms established at their own institutions for diagnosis and treatment.

Figure 1: Lung Cancer Staging: lymph node staging from IASLC 7th edition*

N Regional Lymph Nodes	Definition
N0	No regional lymph node metastasis
N1	Metastasis in ipsilateral peribronchial and/or ipsilateral hilar lymph nodes (including intrapulmonary lymph nodes)
N2	Metastasis in ipsilateral mediastinal and /or subcarinal lymph nodes
N3	Metastasis in contralateral mediastinal or contralateral hilar lymph nodes

* Revised to show changes directly relevant to performance of EBUS-TBNA

Figure 2: Identification and nomenclature of nodal regions

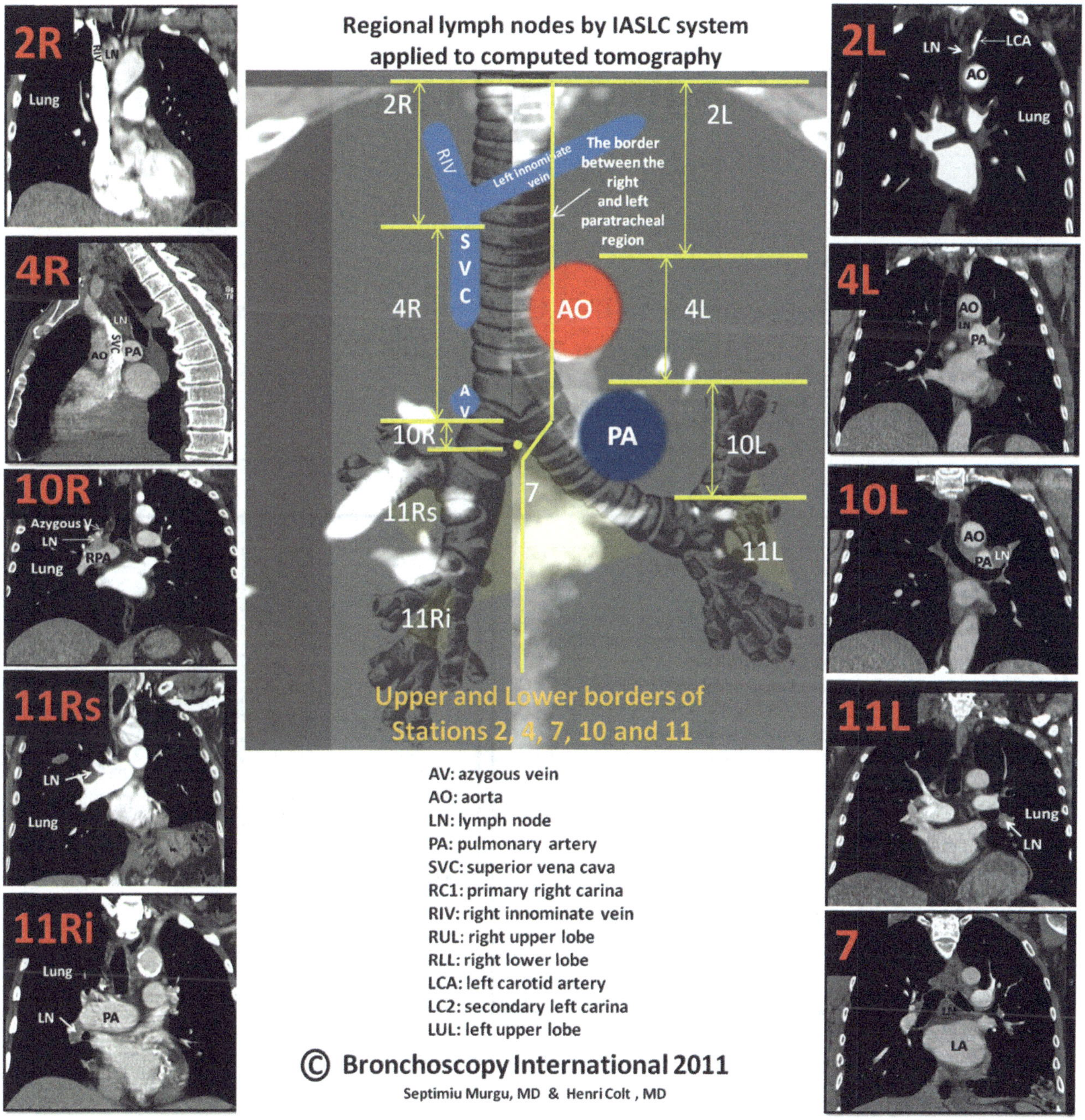

Prognosis, Staging, and Lymph Node Map

Staging according to IASLC 7th edition staging system
(Also in Chest 2009;136:260-271)

IASLC 7th Edition

N (Regional Lymph Nodes)	
NX	Regional lymph nodes cannot be assessed
N0	No regional lymph node metastasis
N1	Metastasis in ipsilateral peribronchial and/or ipsilateral hilar lymph nodes and intrapulmonary nodes, including involvement by direct extension
N2	Metastasis in ipsilateral mediastinal and/or subcarinal lymph node(s)
N3	Metastasis in contralateral mediastinal, contralateral hilar, ipsilateral or contralateral scalene, or supraclavicular lymph node(s)
M (Distant Metastasis)	
MX	Distant metastasis cannot be assessed
M0	No distant metastasis
M1	Distant metastasis
M1a	Separate tumor nodule(s) in a contralateral lobe; tumor with pleural nodules or malignant pleural (or pericardial) effusion[b]
M1b	Distant metastasis

T/M	Subgroup	N0	N1	N2	N3
T1	T1a	Ia	IIa	IIIa	IIIb
	T1b	Ia	IIa	IIIa	IIIb
T2	T2a	Ib	IIa	IIIa	IIIb
	T2b	IIa	IIb	IIIa	IIIb
T3	$T3_{>7}$	IIb	IIIa	IIIa	IIIb
	$T3_{Inv}$	IIb	IIIa	IIIa	IIIb
	$T3_{Satell}$	IIb	IIIa	IIIa	IIIb
T4	$T4_{Inv}$	IIIa	IIIa	IIIb	IIIb
	$T4_{Ipsi\ Nod}$	IIIa	IIIa	IIIb	IIIb
M1	$M1a_{Contra\ Nod}$	IV	IV	IV	IV
	$M1a_{Pl\ Dissem}$	IV	IV	IV	IV
	M1b	IV	IV	IV	IV

Goldstraw P, Crowley J, Chanksy K, Giroux D, Groome P, Rami-Porta R, Postums P, Rusch V, Sobin L. The IASLC Lung Cancer Staging Project: Proposals for the Revision of the TNM Stage Groupings in the Forthcoming (Seventh) Edition of the TNM Classification of Malignant Tumours. J Thorac Oncol 2007: 2; 706-704.

Changes in IASLC 8th Edition (Downloaded from https://www.iaslc.org/research-education/publications-resources-guidelines?title=&resource_category%5B0%5D=929&date=&ver=2019-05-22-154420-317)

IASLC Staging and Prognostic Factors Committee Recommendations Regarding 8th Edition T-Descriptors

Descriptor	7th edition	Proposal for 8th edition
</= 1 cm	T1a	T1a
> 1 - 2 cm	T1a	T1b
> 2 - 3 cm	T1b	T1c
> 3 - 4 cm	T2a	T2a
> 4 - 5 cm	T2a	T2b
> 5 - 7 cm	T2b	T3
> 7 cm	T3	T4
Bronchus < 2 cm	T3	T2
Complete atelectasis/ pneumonitis	T3	T2
Diaphragm invasion	T3	T4
Mediastinal pleura	T3	-

IASLC

From: Rami-Porta R, Bolejack V, Giroux D, et al. The IASLC Lung Cancer Staging Project: The New Database to Inform the Eighth Edition of the TNM Classification of Lung Cancer. *J Thorac Oncol* 2014;9:1618-1624.

CRAB Cancer Research and Biostatistics

IASLC Staging and Prognostic Factors Committee Recommendations Regarding 8th Edition N-Descriptors

- Present N descriptors remain the same
- Quantification of nodal disease is recommended for further study:
  - pN1a: involvement of single pN1 nodal station
  - pN1b: involvement of multiple pN1 nodal stations
  - pN2a1: involvement of single pN2 nodal station without pN1 (skip pN2)
  - pN2a2: involvement of single pN2 nodal station with pN1
  - pN2b: involvement of multiple pN2 nodal stations
  - pN3: as it is

From: Asamura H, Chansky K, Crowley J, et al. The International Association for the Study of Lung Cancer Lung Cancer Staging Project: Proposals for the Revision of the N Descriptors in the Forthcoming 8th Edition of the TNM Classification for Lung Cancer. *J Thorac Oncol* 2015; 10:1675-1684.

IASLC

CRAB Cancer Research and Biostatistics

Changes in IASLC 8th Edition cont.

IASLC Staging and Prognostic Factors Committee Recommendations Regarding 8th Edition M-Descriptors

Descriptor	7th edition	Proposal for 8th edition
Intrathoraic metastasis (pleural/pericardial effusion, contralateral/bilateral tumor nodules, pleural/pericardial nodules)	M1a	M1a
Single extrathoracic metastatic lesion	M1b	M1b
Multiple extrathoracic lesions	M1b	M1c

IASLC

From: Eberhardt WE, Mitchell A, Crowley J, et al. The IASLC Lung Cancer Staging Project: Proposals for the Revision of the M Descriptors in the Forthcoming Eighth Edition of the TNM Classification of Lung Cancer. *J Thorac Oncol* 2015;10:1515–1522.

CRAB Cancer Research And Biostatistics

IASLC Staging and Prognostic Factors Committee Recommendations Regarding 8th Edition Stage Groupings

	N0	N1	N2	N3	M1a any N	M1b any N	M1c any N
T1a	IA1	IIB	IIIA	IIIB	IVA	IVA	IVB
T1b	IA2	IIB	IIIA	IIIB	IVA	IVA	IVB
T1c	IA3	IIB	IIIA	IIIB	IVA	IVA	IVB
T2a	IB	IIB	IIIA	IIIB	IVA	IVA	IVB
T2b	IIA	IIB	IIIA	IIIB	IVA	IVA	IVB
T3	IIB	IIIA	IIIB	IIIC	IVA	IVA	IVB
T4	IIIA	IIIA	IIIB	IIIC	IVA	IVA	IVB

IASLC

From: Goldstraw P, Chansky K, Crowley J, et al. The IASLC Lung Cancer Staging Project: Proposals for Revision of the TNM Stage Groupings in the Forthcoming (Eighth) Edition of the TNM Classification for Lung Cancer. *J Thorac Oncol* 2016;11:39-51.

CRAB Cancer Research And Biostatistics

Downloaded from https://www.iaslc.org/research-education/publications-resources-guidelines?title=&resource_category%5B0%5D=929&date=&ver=2019-05-22-154420-317

Changes in IASLC 8th Edition cont.

Core IASLC Data in Support of Recommendations for Stage Groupings
Overall Survival by Clinical Stage

7th Edition Stage Groupings

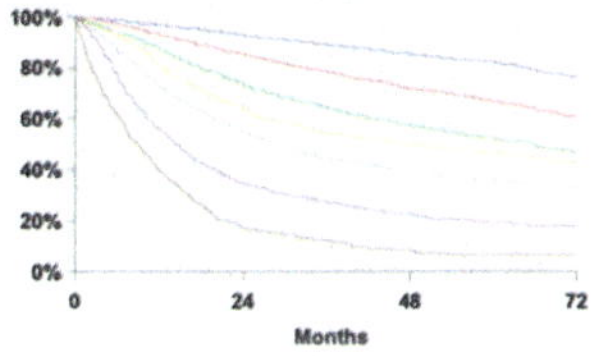

7th Ed.	Events / N	MST	24 Month	60 Month
IA	1119 / 6303	NR	93%	82%
IB	768 / 2492	NR	85%	66%
IIA	424 / 1008	66.0	74%	52%
IIB	382 / 824	49.0	64%	47%
IIIA	2139 / 3344	29.0	55%	36%
IIIB	2101 / 2624	14.1	34%	19%
IV	664 / 882	8.8	17%	6%

Proposed Stage Groupings

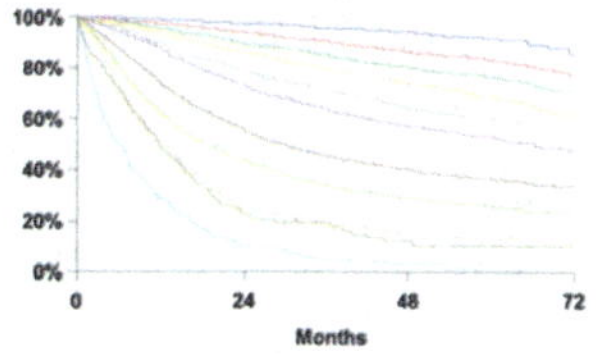

Proposed	Events / N	MST	24 Month	60 Month
IA1	68 / 781	NR	97%	92%
IA2	505 / 3105	NR	94%	83%
IA3	546 / 2417	NR	90%	77%
IB	560 / 1928	NR	87%	68%
IIA	215 / 585	NR	79%	60%
IIB	605 / 1453	66.0	72%	53%
IIIA	2052 / 3200	29.3	55%	36%
IIIB	1551 / 2140	19.0	44%	26%
IIIC	831 / 986	12.6	24%	13%
IVA	336 / 484	11.5	23%	10%
IVB	328 / 398	6.0	10%	0%

- **MST, median survival time.**
- **Survival is weighted by type of database submission: registry versus other.**

IASLC

From: Goldstraw P, Chansky K, Crowley J, et al. The IASLC Lung Cancer Staging Project: Proposals for Revision of the TNM Stage Groupings in the Forthcoming (Eighth) Edition of the TNM Classification for Lung Cancer. *J Thorac Oncol* 2016;11:39-51.

CRAB Cancer Research and Biostatistics

Core IASLC Data in Support of Recommendations for Stage Groupings
Overall Survival by Pathologic Stage

7th Edition Stage Groupings

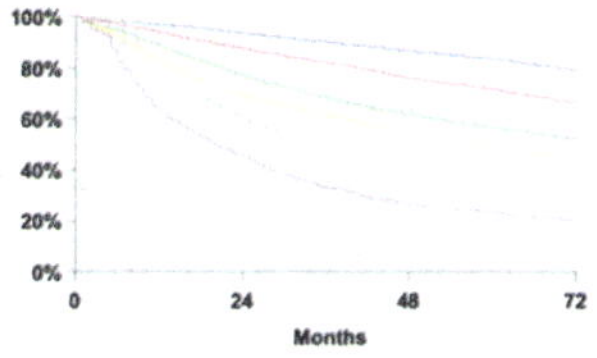

7th Ed.	Events / N	MST	24 Month	60 Month
IA	1837 / 11423	NR	94%	83%
IB	2168 / 7711	NR	87%	71%
IIA	1514 / 3702	NR	77%	57%
IIB	1325 / 2776	58.9	70%	49%
IIIA	3467 / 5818	35.0	61%	36%
IIIB	364 / 506	20.0	45%	23%

Proposed Stage Groupings

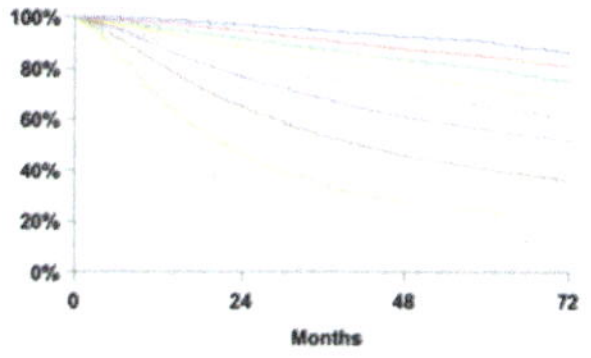

Proposed	Events / N	MST	24 Month	60 Month
IA1	139 / 1389	NR	97%	90%
IA2	823 / 5633	NR	94%	85%
IA3	875 / 4401	NR	92%	80%
IB	1618 / 6095	NR	89%	73%
IIA	556 / 1638	NR	82%	65%
IIB	2175 / 5226	NR	76%	56%
IIIA	3219 / 5756	41.9	65%	41%
IIIB	1215 / 1729	22.0	47%	24%
IIIC	55 / 69	11.0	30%	12%

- **MST, median survival time.**
- **Survival is weighted by type of database submission: registry versus other.**

IASLC

From: Goldstraw P, Chansky K, Crowley J, et al. The IASLC Lung Cancer Staging Project: Proposals for Revision of the TNM Stage Groupings in the Forthcoming (Eighth) Edition of the TNM Classification for Lung Cancer. *J Thorac Oncol* 2016;11:39-51.

CRAB Cancer Research and Biostatistics

Downloaded from https://www.iaslc.org/research-education/publications-resources-guidelines?title=&resource_category%5B0%5D=929&date=&ver=2019-05-22-154420-317

****

EBUS Lymph Node Map (See video): Describes scope and transducer placement

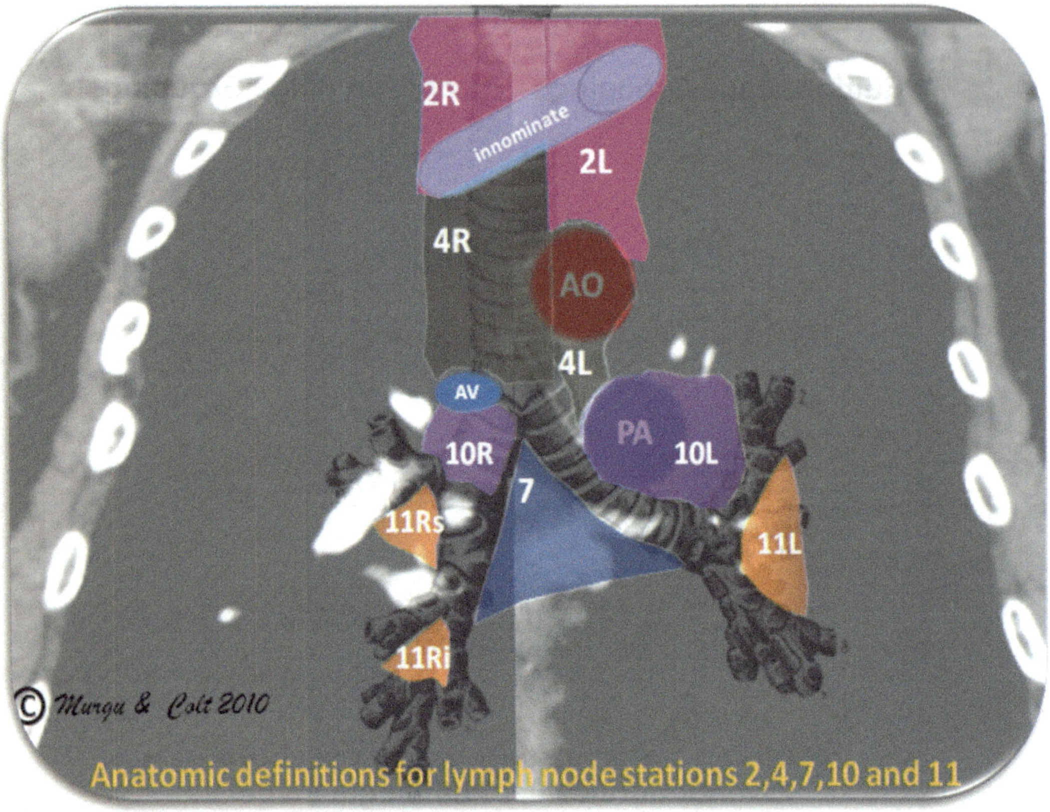

1. **Station 2R**, the upper right paratracheal region, extends across the midline to the left lateral border of the trachea. The upper border is the apex of the right lung and pleural space, and, the upper border of the sternal manubrium. The lower border is at the intersection of the caudal margin of the innominate vein with the trachea. The EBUS probe is placed against the right tracheal wall in the upper trachea at the level of the 4-5th tracheal rings. The transducer is oriented towards the 3-o'clock position.
2. **Station 2L**, the upper left paratracheal region, includes nodes extending to the left of the left lateral border of the trachea. The upper border is the apex of the left lung and pleural space, and in the midline, the upper border of the sternal manubrium. The lower border is the superior aspect of the aortic arch. To visualize this station, the EBUS scope is placed against the left tracheal wall in the upper trachea at the level of the 4-5th tracheal rings. The transducer is oriented towards the 9-o'clock position.
3. **Station 4R**, the right lower paratracheal region, includes right lower paratracheal nodes, and pretracheal nodes extending to the left lateral border of trachea. The upper border is the intersection of the caudal margin of the innominate vein with the trachea. The lower border is the lower margin of the azygos vein. The EBUS scope is placed proximal to the main carina and turned towards the 3-o'clock position. 4R nodes, however, are often pretracheal, in a more anterior position, so the scope may need to be turned counterclockwise towards the 12 o'clock position.

4. **Station 10R** is immediately adjacent to the right main bronchus and hilar vessels, including the proximal portions of the pulmonary veins and main pulmonary artery. The upper border is the lower margin of the azygos vein. The lower border is the interlobar region between the right upper lobe and bronchus intermedius. To visualize this hilar nodal station, the EBUS scope can be gently advanced from the carina to the origin of the right upper lobe bronchus. The transducer is oriented antero-laterally towards the 2-o'clock position.
5. **Station 7** is subcarinal. The upper border of this region is the main carina of the trachea. Its lower borders are the distal end of the bronchus intermedius on the right, and the upper border of the lower lobe bronchus on the left. The scope is placed in the proximal right or left main bronchus. The transducer is oriented medially.
6. **Station 4L** includes nodes to the left of the left lateral border of the trachea, medial to the ligamentum arteriosum. Its upper border is the upper margin of the aortic arch. Its lower border is the upper margin of the left main pulmonary artery. The scope is placed in the proximal left main bronchus at the level of main carina. The scope is turned to the left, towards the 9-o'clock position.
7. **Station 10L** is immediately adjacent to the left main bronchus and hilar vessels, including the proximal portions of the pulmonary veins and main pulmonary artery. The upper border is the upper margin of the left pulmonary artery. The lower border is the interlobar region between the left upper and lower lobes. The EBUS scope is placed in the proximal left upper lobe bronchus. The tip of the scope is pressed to the bronchial wall towards the 11-o'clock position.
8. **Station 11L** is comprised of nodes located in the region between the origins of the left upper and lower lobar bronchi. The scope is advanced towards the proximal part of the lower lobe bronchus. The transducer is oriented laterally towards the left in order to scan for interlobar lymph nodes.
9. **Station 11R superior** includes nodes between the right upper lobe bronchus and the bronchus intermedius. The tip of the EBUS scope is placed in the proximal bronchus intermedius, just below the subcarina separating the upper lobe bronchus from the bronchus intermedius. The area between the 2-o'clock and 4-o'clock positions is scanned.
10. **Station 11R inferior** is between the middle lobe and right lower lobe bronchi. The EBUS scope is positioned in the proximal right lower lobe bronchus. The transducer can then be oriented towards the right lateral wall.

****

EBUS-CT-White Light Bronchoscopy: Synopsis

The purpose of this synopsis is to provide the reader with a brief overview of EBUS-CT-White light bronchoscopy correlations in order to enhance procedural strategy and planning. A poster is provided so that EBUS bronchoscopists might familiarize themselves with radiographic anatomic landmarks and their EBUS/white light bronchoscopy correlates. Readers are encouraged to study the instructional video for further information, and to discuss procedural planning strategies and techniques with colleagues and EBUS experts. This is just one example of how imaging studies can be used to help plan EBUS-TBNA. Readers are encouraged to develop and discuss other methodologies with their peers.

See Poster in your curriculum booklet as well as video

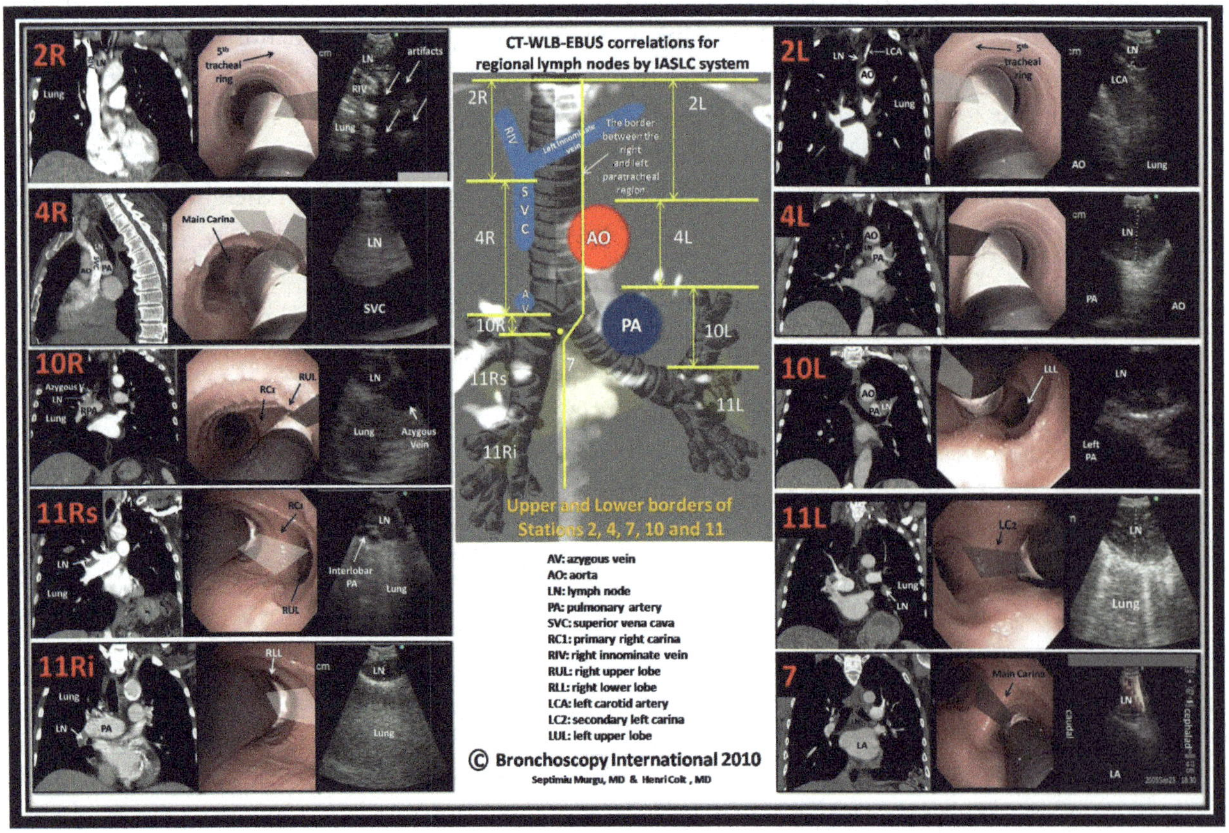

1. Specific Computed Tomography views, primarily the coronal views, can help plan an EBUS procedure. In this example we shall use the lower paratracheal station 4L limited by the superior margin of the aortic arch and the upper rim of the left main pulmonary artery. The lymph node is usually located lateral to the trachea at the level of the main carina.
2. The bronchoscope is placed in the lower trachea, approximately at the origin of the left main bronchus. With the balloon inflated, the transducer is turned towards the left to visualize the left paratracheal region. Station 4L is ALWAYS to the left of the left lateral border of the trachea.
3. The coronal computed tomography view correlates well with this EBUS scanning plane. The aortic arch is seen proximal, and the left pulmonary artery is seen distal to the lymph node. Actually, the EBUS image is projected on the monitor as if the scope were horizontal. The green dot on the monitor represents the point where the needle exits the scope. This corresponds to the cephalad aspect of the body. This dot is by default, towards the 1'o'clock position on the monitor.
4. Several adjustments can be made to the coronal CT image in order to bring the scope to a horizontal position and the green dot cephalad (towards the 1 o'clock position on the monitor) to match the EBUS image.
5. Rotate the CT image clockwise in order to bring the scope to a horizontal position and the green dot towards 1 o'clock. Because the green dot is cephalad, the vascular structure at 3'o'clock is proximal and represents the aorta, while the vascular structure at 9'o'clock is more distal and represents the left pulmonary artery.

****

EBUS Physics and Terminology: Synopsis

Ultrasound (US) is an imaging modality based on the reflective properties of sound waves. Ultrasonography thus represents mechanical energy that causes compression and rarefaction of a conducting material or substance known as medium. This technology uses sound waves with frequencies of 20kHz or higher, inaudible to humans[1].

Echogenicity represents the extent to which a tissue or substance gives rise to reflections of ultrasonic waves. When US images are displayed on a gray scale, the strongest echo signal is white, and when no sound wave is reflected, the image is black or in ultrasound terms, anechoic (Figure 1). The intensity of the signal determining echogenicity depends on the reflected wave amplitude. The terms used in ultrasonography to describe a certain tissue or structure include: isoechoic, comparable with the surrounding tissue; hypoechoic, weaker than the surrounding tissue and hyperechoic, stronger than the surrounding tissue (Figure 1).

Frequency and Wavelength represent a specific number of vibration cycles per second (measured in units of hertz). Endoscopic US frequencies are in the range of 5-30 MHz[2]. Current dedicated EBUS-TBNA bronchoscopes allow changes in frequency from 5 to12 MHz. The wavelength of US represents the distance between two successive pulses: the higher the frequency, the shorter the related wavelength.

Propagation is the process through which sound advances through various tissues. The transducer sends out a brief pulse of sound that penetrates the tissue. The sound waves are reflected back to a transducer, which serves as the sensor and source of signal. US is reflected at tissue boundaries and interfaces, like light off a mirror (Figure 1); it reflects very well wherever there is a significant change in the propagation medium. The degree of **reflection** is determined by the acoustic impedance of the adjacent tissue, largely related to tissue density. When the US beam strikes an interface, it undergoes refraction, scattering, and attenuation as it passes through tissue, all of which degrade image quality on examining deeper structures (Figure 1).

---

[1] Kurimoto N. Diagnosis of depth penetration in the tracheobronchial tree. In: Kurimoto N (ed.). Endobronchial Ultrasonography. Kinpodo, Kyoto, 2001; pp 33–38. Also, see Greenleaf JF. ABCs of Ultrasound Imaging. In: Ernst A, Feller-Kopman D (eds). Ultrasound Guided Procedures and Investigations. A manual for the clinician. Taylor & Francis, New York, 2006; pp 1-16

[2] Nishina K, Hirooka K, Wiegand J, Dremel H. Principles and Practice of endoscopic ultrasound. In Bolliger CT et al (eds): Clinical Chest Ultrasound: From the ICU to the bronchoscopy suite. Prog Respir Res. Basel, Karger, 2009, vol 37,pp 110-127

Refraction represents a change in direction of the incident US beam, while **scattering** is the spread of the US beam in different directions.

Attenuation is the loss of energy caused by absorption (when the vibration of the US wave is converted to heat due to friction). Attenuation depends on the medium, being much higher in air than in water and on the frequency, increasing with higher frequencies (Figure 1). The bigger the difference in acoustic properties between two media, the larger the proportion of reflected US and the smaller the transmitted US. Such an acoustic interface results in a strong echo signal (i.e., lung tissue or air in the bronchial system) (Figure 1); the lower the density, the higher the attenuation (i.e. higher attenuation in air than in water) (Figure 1).

Penetration refers to the distance between an imaged area and the transducer. The time delay between the energy entering the tissue and returning to the US transducer determines the depth from which the signal arises (longer times equal greater depths since depth=velocity X time/2). Large transducers that transmit powerful beams will increase penetration depth (it goes without saying, therefore, that penetration depth is less in EBUS than in thoracic US) (Figure 1). The maximum penetration depth depends on the frequency used: higher frequencies (i.e., 20 MHz) do not penetrate as deep as the lower frequencies (7.5 MHz). Thus, superficial structures are better visualized with higher frequency and deeper structures with lower frequency transducers. For these reasons, in bronchoscopy, the 20 MHz EBUS radial probe can be used for imaging airway wall layers, while the 7.5 MHz is used for visualizing deeper structures such as lymph nodes and blood vessels (Figure 1).

Resolution refers to the level of detail of an image; it is the capacity of a system to distinguish small objects from others and is determined by the frequency and duration of the transmitted sound phase. Resolution is categorized in two types: axial, representing the ability to resolve objects within the imaging plane at different depths, and lateral, representing the ability to resolve objects in the imaging plane that are located side by side.

Image Artifacts are due to image distortion caused by normal phenomena of refraction, scattering and attenuation which may interfere with the ability to properly identify an US target (i.e., lymph node, blood vessel). Yet, image artifacts can be useful because they help describe the properties of tissues (i.e., calcification or necrosis within a lymph node). Understanding the different types of artifacts helps us identify and obtain a clear image of a real target and perform a safe needle aspiration without puncturing vascular structures or lung parenchyma. Common types of artifacts seen during EBUS imaging include reverberation and attenuation artifacts.

- Reverberation artifacts occur when a highly reflective tissue is parallel to the transducer, such as when the water filled balloon of the EBUS probe/scope is not in contact with the airway wall, and the US waves are repeatedly reflected between the tissue surface (airway wall) and the transducer[2]. The resulting effect is strong false echoes appearing as multiple equally spaced lines on the ultrasound image (Figure 2).

---

[3] Nishina K, Hirooka K, Wiegand J, Dremel H. Principles and Practice of endoscopic ultrasound. In Boliger CT et al (eds): Clinical Chest Ultrasound: From the ICU to the bronchoscopy suite. Prog Respir Res. Basel, Karger, 2009, vol 37, pp 110-127

- Attenuation artifacts are comprised of the tadpole tail sign **and** the acoustic shadow. Tissues with low acoustic impedance (i.e., necrotic lymph nodes, mediastinal cysts) result in lower attenuation than tissues with higher impedance. For the tadpole tail artifact, the echo at the distal border of the low impedance structure will be higher and US will display the area distal to the low impedance structure more brightly compared to the surrounding tissue (Figure 2). The acoustic shadow artifact is exactly the reverse of the tadpole tail as the area behind a high impedance structure is displayed with lower brightness than the rest of the surrounding tissue. Since the US beam is almost completely reflected at the border or attenuated within the high impedance structure, the posterior area does not receive US waves and appears as a hypoechoic shadow (Figure 2).

Figure 1: Ultrasound terminology and principles

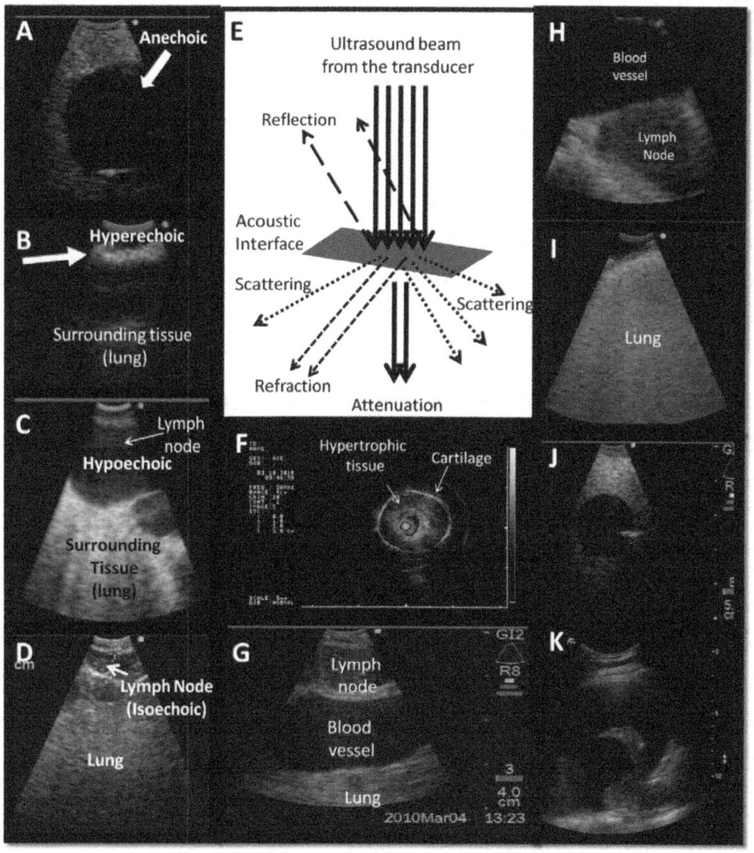

Figure 1 Legend. Principles and terminology of ultrasound: (A). A structure (i.e., blood vessel) which does not reflect the sound waves at all is termed anechoic. (B). A hyperechoic pattern (i.e., cartilaginous nodule in tracheopathica osteochondroplastica) occurs when the echoes are stronger than those of the surrounding tissues. (C). A hypoechoic structure (i.e., lymph node) occurs when the echoes are weaker than those from the surrounding tissues. (D). This lymph node is labeled isoechoic, because the echoes are of comparable amplitude with the surrounding tissue (i. e. lung). (E). The US beam undergoes reflection, refraction, scattering, and attenuation as it passes through tissue; all of these degrade image quality on examining deeper structures but the last three processes cause the US waves reflected back to the transducer to be much weaker. (F). Increased attenuation and low penetration depth occur when structures are visualized

with high frequency probes: the hypertrophic stenotic tissue and the intact cricoid cartilage are clearly visualized, but the deeper structures are not when the 20 MHz radial probe is used. (G). When the curved linear EBUS transducer with 7.5 MHz frequency is used the attenuation is decreased, the penetration depth is increased and the EBUS image shows the right lower paratracheal lymph node, the superior vena cava and the distal normal lung parenchyma but details of the airway wall structures cannot be assessed. (H). Attenuation also depends on the medium, being low in fluid (i.e., blood vessels). (I). Attenuation is high in air (i.e., normal lung tissue). (J). The depth of penetration is also directly dependent on the size of the transducer. A relatively superficial penetration (i.e., 5 cm) is achieved using the small EBUS curved linear transducer. (K). A deep penetration (i.e., 15 cm) can be obtained by using large thoracic transducers.

Figure 2: Image artifacts

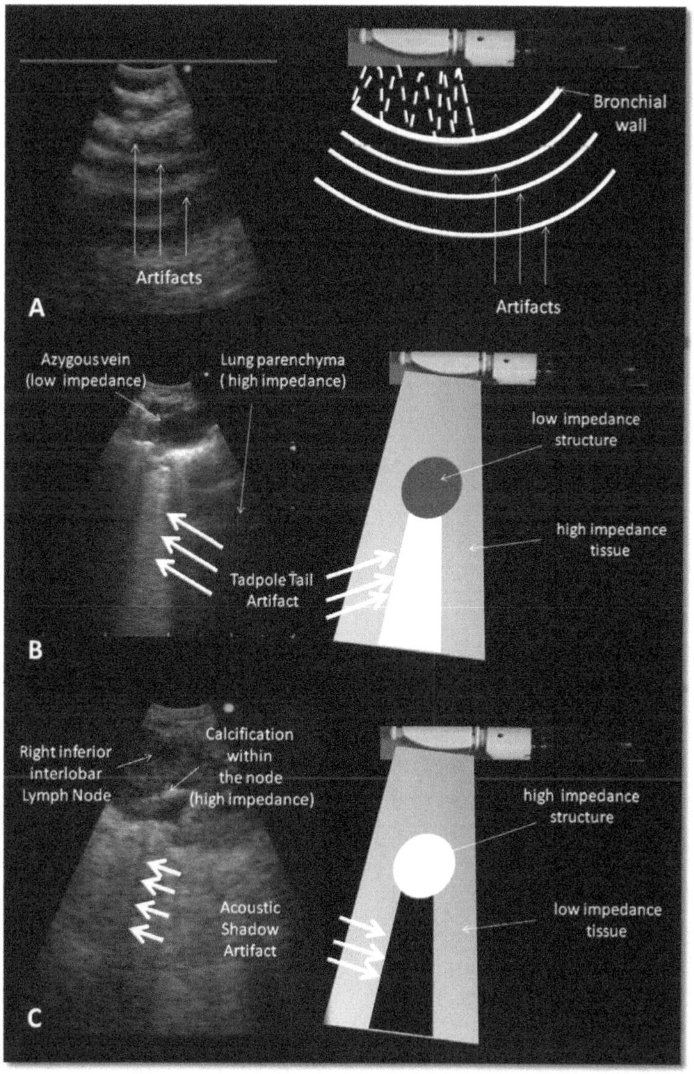

Figure 2 Legend. Image artifacts. (A). Reverberation artifacts: when the water filled balloon of the EBUS bronchoscope is not in intimate contact with the airway wall, the US waves are repeatedly reflected between the highly reflective tissue surface (airway wall) and the transducer; the resulting effect is that strong

false echoes appear as multiple equally spaced lines on the ultrasound image. (B). In the tadpole tail artifact, the echo at the distal border of the low impedance structure (i.e., azygous vein) will be higher and US will display the area distal to the low impedance structure more brightly compared to the surrounding tissue (thick arrows). (C). The acoustic shadow artifact is the reverse effect of the tadpole tail; the area behind a high impedance structure (i.e., calcification within the lymph node) is displayed with lower brightness than the rest of the surrounding tissue. The US beam is attenuated within the high impedance structure and the posterior area appears as a hypoechoic shadow (thick arrows).

****

Moderate Sedation: Synopsis

The purpose of this synopsis is to provide the reader with a brief overview of moderate sedation as it might apply to flexible bronchoscopy. It is assumed that institutions and practitioners have different biases and regulations. Herein a short summary is provided so that beginner bronchoscopists might acquire at least some of the elements necessary for a safe procedure. Readers are encouraged to follow guidelines and protocols established in their own institutions.

Definitions

- Moderate sedation may be produced by the use of intravenous, oral, transmucosal or intramuscular narcotics, sedatives or anxiolytic medications
- Moderate sedation is a medically controlled state of depressed consciousness that allows protective reflexes to be maintained, while retaining the patient's ability to maintain a patent airway independently and continuously. This implies that the patient is mildly drowsy but arouses to voice easily. This is to be distinguished from
- Deep sedation, where the patient is arousable only by vigorous stimulation and may lose the ability to maintain airway patency and protection.

ASA Classification

- ASA 1: normal and healthy patient
- ASA 2: Mild controlled systemic disease and no functional limitation
- ASA 3: Moderate to severe systemic disease that limits activity.
- ASA 4: severe systemic disease that is a constant threat to life or is functionally incapacitating.
- ASA 5: Moribund and not expected to survive without surgery

Equipment

- Informed consent for sedation should be obtained in addition to consent for the procedure.
- Oximetry

- Ability to monitor the patient for vital signs, airway patency, degree of wakefulness.
- Electrocardiogram
- Intravenous access
- Rescue equipment for any patient moving into deep sedation, including crash cart and defibrillator
- Appropriate size endotracheal tubes and ability to ventilate patient (including self-inflating Ambu-bag and mask system) should be available.
- Reversal agents for narcotics and benzodiazepines
- Charting should include baseline ventilatory, hemodynamic, neurologic status, time of administration of medication, dose administered, type of medication used, physical examination, informed consent, allergies, nothing to eat 8 hours prior to the procedure (except for clear liquids and medications, up to four hours prior to procedure).
- Ability to monitor patient status at least every 15 minutes during the procedure and for a minimum of thirty (30) minutes after the procedure and/or until patient returns to baseline status, including pulse oximetry equal or greater than 92% on room air, or assured with supplemental oxygen if patient on oxygen.
- Following administration of reversal agents such as naloxone, patient should not be discharged for a minimum of one (1) hour, and flumazenil two (2) hours.

Potential contraindications

- Uncooperative patients
- Mentally ill patients
- Severe cardiac, pulmonary, hepatic, renal or central nervous disease
- Pregnancy
- Morbid obesity
- Alcohol or drug abuse
- History of sleep apnea

High risk patients

- Previous problems with anesthesia or sedation
- Previous surgery or radiation or injury to neck or face
- Stridor, snoring, or sleep apnea
- Dysmorphic facial features
- Advanced rheumatoid arthritis
- Significant obesity, protruding teeth
- Small mouth opening (<3cm in adults), macroglossia, non-visible uvula, tonsillar hypertrophy, short neck, limited neck extension, decreased hyoid-mental distance (<3cm in adult).

Response to complications

- Ability to rotate patient onto lateral decubitus position in case of vomiting.
- Ability to insert a nasal trumpet
- Ability to perform chin lift/neck extension in case of obstructed airway
- Oral suction should always be available
- Ability to establish a safe and patent airway, and provide hemodynamic and circulatory support in case of compromise.

Specific medications

- *Midazolam* (Versed) is currently the most widely used agent for moderate sedation and anxiolysis. It is a water-soluble benzodiazepine with rapid onset of action. It is four times more potent on a mg per mg basis than
  - When administered intravenously, sedation and anxiolysis usually occurs within 2 minutes. Complete recovery of motor performance and consciousness occurs within one hour in most individuals.
  - Combining Midazolam and opioides increases the incidence of apnea. Large doses can produce prolonged drowsiness and cardio-respiratory arrest. Central nervous system dysfunction, including confusion and seizures can be seen in patients with brain metastases and paraneoplastic syndromes.
  - Ventilation is depressed by 0.15 mg/kg, especially in patients with COPD. The peak effect of respiratory depression occurs at three minutes following injection and remains for approximately 15 minutes. It can be most pronounced in geriatric and COPD patients.
- *Fentanyl* is a synthetic opiate analog that is structurally different from morphine or meperidine. It is 100 times more potent than morphine. The usual adult dose is 50-100 micrograms. Given intravenously, its onset of action and maximum respiratory depression effect occurs about 5-10 minutes after administration, and lasts 30-60 minutes.
  - Given intramuscularly, the onset of action is within 7-15 minutes with duration of action lasting up to two hours.
  - Fentanyl should never be used in patients receiving MAO inhibitors because of increased risk of respiratory depression and coma.
- *Combination drugs.* Sedative responses are increased in patients who have received opioides or other benzodiazepines. Level of sedation and risk for respiratory depression are increased in the elderly and in patients with pre-existing respiratory dysfunction.
- *Reversal agents*:
  - Naloxone is a pure opiate antagonist that reverses all effects and side effects of opiates). The initial dose is 0.1-0.2 mg IV, SQ, IM or via endotracheal tube and can be repeated every 2 minutes. The onset of action is about 30 seconds. Actually, no more than 0.4 mg should be administered because this might lead to increased activity of the sympathetic nervous system from acute termination of analgesia. Consequently, patients may develop hypertension, dysrhythmias, and pulmonary edema.

- Flumazenil is a benzodiazepine antagonist that should be administered (0.2 mg IV over 15 seconds, then repeated every minute up to a maximum of 1 mg). Low doses of Flumazenil will reliably reverse sedation within 2 minutes, but higher doses are needed to reverse benzodiazepine-related anxiolysis. Duration of action is about 60 minutes. Side effects include nausea, vomiting, tremors, seizures, tears and dizziness. Contrary to naloxone, it does not cause hemodynamic instability.

Dosing guidelines

- *Midazolam* single dose 1 mg IV, onset of action 1-2.5 minutes, total dose 5 mg
- *Lorazapam* single dose 2 mg IV, onset of action 20-30 minutes, total dose 4 mg
- *Morphine* single dose 2-4 mg IV, onset of action 1-5 minutes, total dose 10 mg
- *Fentanyl* single dose 50 mcg IV, onset of action 1-5 min, total dose 100 mcg

****

SECTION 3

Tumor Markers and EBUS*

1. *Tumor Markers:* Synopsis with instructional video.
2. *Clinical pathway: tumor markers in advanced NSCLC.* Module with instructional specimen handling videos.

* Checklists, videos, and post-tests used at the discretion of program director. Videos viewable on You Tube (BronchOrg site) and through www.Bronchoscopy.org.

Tumor Markers: Synopsis

The purpose of this synopsis is to provide readers with a brief overview of tumor markers. Lung cancer is increasingly recognized as a heterogeneous disease. Therapeutic empiricism based on tumor histology is therefore being replaced by therapeutic strategies that integrate individual clinical, cytohistologic and molecular parameters. Using these strategies, lung cancer treatment is increasingly personalized, and several biomarkers are showing promise as prognostic and predictive parameters in NSCLC, independent of disease stage, patient performance status or gender. This synopsis summarizes some of these contributions to personalized lung cancer treatment, describes several assay technologies used for biomarker analysis potentially pertinent to bronchoscopic needle aspiration, and encourage the formation of multidisciplinary teams dedicated to the science and applications of personalized therapy. The synopsis includes

- EBUS-TBNA and molecular marker analysis for NSCLC synopsis
- A glossary of terms
- An example of a clinical pathway exercise pertaining to TBNA and tumor markers

EBUS-TBNA and Molecular Analysis for NSCLC Synopsis*

Introduction

A majority of patients with lung cancer are diagnosed using small volume specimens obtained by biopsy or needle aspiration, particularly if patients present with suspected advanced disease. Staging and restaging is also performed in this fashion. The role of EBUS-TBNA is increasing for these purposes, and often, may be the *only* source of material obtained. Furthermore, in this era of personalized medicine, treatment decisions are being made based on a patient's molecular tumor profile, which also has a role in determining prognosis. Patients with lung cancer, now recognized as a heterogeneous collection of diseases with diverse molecular characteristics, even within a single histologic type such as adenocarcinoma (1), are thus increasingly treated based on matching drug profiles with specific mutations of a patient's tumor (2).

The objectives of this synopsis are:

1. To describe the *rationale* for using molecular markers for targeting therapy in patients with NSCLC.
2. To describe specific *molecular predictors* of response or resistance to targeted therapy and chemotherapy[1].
3. To describe the *assay technologies* for molecular biomarker analysis pertinent to EBUS-TBNA specimens.
4. To describe *specimen selection, handling* after EBUS-TBNA, and sample preparation for molecular testing.
5. To describe *molecular analysis-based strategies* for NSCLC using EBUS-TBNA samples.
6. To provide a *glossary* of key terms used in molecular biology and in this synopsis.

* *This synopsis has been prepared by Dr. Septimiu Murgu carefully edited by Dr. Henri Colt*

[1] Personalized therapy includes what is often referred to as "targeted therapy" (e.g. the effect of monoclonal antibodies and small molecules targeting EGFR), and chemotherapy (which may be adjusted based on predictive molecular markers). The National Cancer Institute defines targeted therapy as the administration of drugs or other substances that block the growth and spread of cancer by interfering with specific molecules involved in tumor growth and progression (downloaded 8/24/2011, http://www.cancer.gov/cancertopics/factsheet/Therapy/targeted).

Rationale for Using Molecular Markers for Individualized NSCLC Treatment.

- Several molecules have potential utility as prognostic[2] and predictive[3] parameters in NSCLC, independent of disease stage, patient performance status or gender. These include genes such as ERCC1 and RRM1 involved in nucleotide metabolism and DNA damage repair, epidermal growth factor receptor (EGFR) involved in cell proliferation and survival, and oligonucleotide expression array profiles, which are signatures of gene expression associated with specific tumor phenotypes.
- The introduction of targeted therapy and the discovery of predictive and prognostic markers have thus become a focus of individualized or personalized care for patients with NSCLC.
- Targeted therapy is highly dependent on which pathway is activated for a particular tumor.[4]
- Recent genomic studies in adenocarcinoma of the lung identified other mutations in tyrosine kinase genes including KRAS, NRAS, BRAF, PI3KCA, and others in frequencies exceeding 1% (3, 4, 5, 6).

Specific Molecular Predictors of Response or Resistance to Personalized Therapy

ERCC1 (Excision-repair cross-complementation group 1)

- This protein participates in the nucleotide excision repair process responsible for the repair of platinum-induced DNA damage (8).
- ERCC1 may be a predictor for platinum resistance in advanced NSCLC; high levels (high expression of ERCC1 mRNA) in NSCLC tumors predict longer survival in patients randomized to treatment without chemotherapy (control group) and a lower likelihood of response to platinum-based chemotherapy (9).
- While immunohistochemical (IHC) staining can be used to determine expression of ERCC1 (10), many studies report using RT-PCR on specimens that are frozen or preserved in formalin.

RRM1 (Regulatory subunit 1 of ribonucleotide reducatase)

- Ribonucleotide reductase is an enzyme involved in DNA synthesis and repair. This enzyme catalyzes the biosynthesis of deoxyribonucleotides from corresponding ribonucleotides; RRM1, the regulatory subunit of ribonucleotide reductase, plays a role in suppressing tumor cell migration and metastasis.
- RRM1 gene expression may impact long-term survival independent of stage, performance status, and weight loss (11).

---

[2] This term refers specifically to a marker used for estimating a patient's prognosis (outcome) independent of therapeutic decisions.

[3] This term refers to a marker/parameter that is used to make therapeutic decisions (i.e. the effect of treatment is different in marker-positive and -negative patients).

[4] For example, erlotinib targets EGFR signaling, sorafenib, the ras/raf signaling, vandetanib, the VEGF and EGFR signaling and bexarotene, the retinoid X receptor signaling (7).

- RRM1 mRNA expression is a molecular marker that has been used to customize chemotherapy and improve outcome in lung cancer patients.
    - It is the molecular target of gemcitabine, an antimetabolite with activity in NSCLC and other malignancies.
    - Low RRM1 mRNA expression correlates with increased overall survival in patients receiving gemcitabine/cisplatin (12, 13).
- RRM1 gene expression is detected by IHC or RT-PCR on fresh-frozen and formalin-fixed, paraffin-embedded tumor specimens.

TS (Thymidylate synthase)

- This enzyme involved in DNA biosynthesis (14) is responsible for maintaining intracellular levels of thymidine, important for DNA synthesis and repair.
- TS expression (mRNA) is correlated with resistance to pemetrexed. It is higher in patients with squamous cell carcinoma compared to adenocarcinoma (15).
- TS expression is detected by IHC or RT-PCR on fresh-frozen and formalin-fixed, paraffin-embedded tumor specimens.

EGFR (Epidermal growth factor receptor)

- EGFR is a growth promoting protein lying within the cytoplasmic membrane; its external domain binds growth factors and is the target of large monoclonal antibody drugs such as cetuximab while the internal domain, including the tyrosine kinase domain, is the target of small molecule drugs, known as tyrosine kinase inhibitors (TKIs).
- EGFR gene mutations[5], protein over-expression, and increased gene copy number are biomarkers of response to EGFR inhibitors (16).
- EGFR mutation is most common in lung adenocarcinoma. It is an independent predictor of thyrosine kinase inhibitors (TKI) gefitinib and erlotinib response and survival in patients of advanced NSCLC (17).
- TKI administration is used as first-line therapy for EGFR mutant tumors: only 70%-80% of EGFR mutation-positive tumors, however, will have meaningful responses (18).
- Patients with mutation-negative adenocarcinomas have superior responses to conventional chemotherapy than to TKI administration (18), further demonstrating the importance of using mutational status to guide drug selection.
- EGFR mutation analysis is feasible in needle biopsy/aspiration paraffin-fixed specimens, although they are generally identified by sequence analysis of PCR-amplified exons in which the activating mutations are frequently found.

[5] Mutations in EGFR exons 18-21 occur in the majority. These are usually deletions in exon 19 and point mutations in exon 21 (19). High EGFR copy number occurs in 30% to 50% of NSCLC patients, whereas gene amplification occurs in approximately 10% (20).

- Cytology slides from patients with NSCLC are used to determine EGFR mutation status by PCR (extraction of DNA), high resolution melt analysis (HRMAA), and sequencing;
    - In one study using a PCR technique, the overall specimen insufficiency rate for EBUS was 4%. This was lower than CT guided biopsy. Similar insufficiency rates were observed in smears and cell-block sections (21).
- Mutation analyses can be performed by sequencing-based detection from formalin-fixed paraffin-embedded tissues obtained by biopsy, resection, or using commercially available PCR tests. The percentage of missed mutations seems too high (>30 %) to recommend the use of mutation-specific PCR for diagnostic applications (22).
- EGFR mutation is detected in 10-37% of EBUS-TBNA specimens; EGFR could be analyzed in 98% of cases. EGFR mutations were noted in 27% of patients using the peptide nucleic acid-locked nucleic acid PCR clamp method (23, 24, 25).
- EGFR protein over-expression and increased gene copy number are less consistent predictors of benefit from targeted therapy compared with EGFR mutation status (14). EGFR IHC and FISH testing is performed for these purposes.
    - Cetuximab may benefit patients with advanced NSCLC EGFR positive by IHC (14).
    - Patients with high EGFR gene copy number by EGFR FISH testing benefit from treatment with EGFR inhibitors (improved time to disease progression and performance status).

KRAS (Kristen-Rous sarcoma gene)

- KRAS is a GTP binding protein involved in the G-protein coupled receptor signaling.
- Mutations in the KRAS gene, located downstream of EGFR in its signaling cascade, are in general mutually exclusive with EGFR mutations.
- KRAS gene mutation may be a predictor for resistance to TKIs therapy in patients with NSCLC (26) and be a prognostic marker (27).
- KRAS mutation is detected by PCR technology followed by capillary electrophoresis on 10% neutral buffered formalin fixed paraffin embedded tissue._
- KRAS gene mutations are detected by DNA sequencing in 3.5-7% of EBUS-TBNA specimens (23); Needle sampling is currently considered insufficiently sensitive because resected specimens show the mutation at higher frequencies (~11%). The optimal methodology for the detection of KRAS mutation for needle biopsied samples is uncertain at this time.

P53 gene (tumor protein 53)

- Detected by direct sequencing p53 gene mutations in 41.6% of patients with NSCLC who underwent EBUS-TBNA (23)
- P53 over-expression is associated with chemoresistance in lymph node samples obtained by EBUS-TBNA (28).

EML4-ALK (Echinoderm microtubule-associated protein-like 4 -anaplastic lymphoma kinase)

- The EML4-ALK fusion oncogene results from a small inversion within chromosome 2p. This leads to expression of a chimeric tyrosine kinase, in which the N-terminal half of echinoderm microtubule-associated protein-like 4 (EML4) is fused to the intracellular kinase domain of anaplastic lymphoma kinase (ALK).

- In most cases, ALK rearrangements are non-overlapping with other oncogenic mutations found in NSCLC (i.e. EGFR mutations, KRAS mutations, etc.)
- The potent oncogenic activity of this aberrant molecule can be effectively blocked by small molecular inhibitors that target ALK (29).
    - o Patients with advanced NSCLC whose tumors harbor EML4-ALK fusion genes and who are treated with the ALK TKI crizotinib have high response rates and long progression-free survival times similar to those of patients with NSCLC and EGFR mutations who are treated with erlotinib (30, 31).
- EBUS-TBNA can be used to obtain mediastinal and hilar nodal tissue for multimodal analysis of ALK fusion genes in NSCLC (32).
- Methods for the detection of ALK fusion genes in EBUS-TBNA specimens include IHC, reverse transcription-PCR (RT-PCR) and fluorescent in situ hybridization (FISH) using a minimum of 2 ml of special media for fine needle aspirations or 10% neutral buffered formalin fixed paraffin embedded tissue. Bronchoscopists should discuss media use with their respective pathology departments and/or laboratories doing tumor marker analyses.
- Screening specimens with IHC revealed ALK positivity in 6.4% of cases, all of which possessed echinoderm microtubule–associated protein-like 4–ALK fusion genes detected by FISH and RT-PCR(32).

BRAF

- This protein affects cell division and differentiation.
- Mutations in the BRAF gene, which lies downstream from EGFR, and is required for RAS activation, are seen in 2.5-3% of patients with NSCLC (more common in melanomas) (33).
- An oral inhibitor to mutated BRAF improves outcome in melanoma (34).
- Can be detected by EBUS-TBNA specimens by direct sequencing techniques (35).

Assay Technologies for Molecular Biomarker Analysis

EBUS-TBNA specimens are processed for histologic diagnosis, staging, and molecular marker analysis using the following specific tests

- o *Routine cytology and histology:* slides and tissue block of tumor
- o *IHC:* tissue block; cytology if cell block or extra smears are available
- o *FISH*: tissue block; cytology if cell block or extra smears are available
- o *Mutation analysis*: tissue block; cytology if cell block or extra smears are available

In the following paragraphs a few techniques a described.

Immunohistochemistry (IHC):

- Semi-quantitative method for estimating protein expression; performed at the same time as histologic diagnosis.
- Uses antibodies to detect the presence of specific proteins in cells; antibody based detection may yield inconsistent results because of a variety of factors including a variation in the antibody type, staining protocols, scoring methods and cutoff criteria (14)

Fluorescence in situ hybridization (FISH)

- Detects genomic and chromosomal changes by hybridizing labeled DNA probes to a sample;
- The method uses fluorescently labeled DNA probes that bind ('hybridize') to specific parts of chromosomes and are visualized by fluorescence microscopy.
- used to detect increased gene (i.e. EGFR) copy number and ALK gene rearrangement

Direct Sequencing

- Method for detecting gene mutations; performed by DNA sequencing using a variety of mutation specific commercially available kits.

Gene expression profiles

- Derived from microarrays; reveal genomic signatures; composites of 3-64 genes.
- May be more accurate predictors of tumor recurrence than disease stage, tumor size, nodal status, age, sex, histology or smoking history (36).
- May be used to determine the selection of adjuvant chemotherapy; patients with resected tumors and low risk signatures could be spared additional chemotherapy while patients with high risk signatures could be offered adjuvant chemotherapy.

Specimen Selection, Handling and Sample preparation and for Molecular Testing

- **Rational and limitations of specimen selection for molecular testing:** A major challenge in molecular analysis is to obtain adequate tumor material at the time of diagnostic biopsies to ensure successful testing.
    - o As of this writing (Summer 2011), a firm pathologic diagnosis is a first priority[6]. Cytology specimens that qualify for molecular testing should contain at least 40% tumor cells, a threshold recommended by molecular diagnostics laboratory.
    - o The majority of patients with NSCLC are diagnosed with advanced, non- surgical disease. Detailed descriptions of cytology specimen preparations are reviewed elsewhere (21).

[6] For instance, immunostains for thyroid transcription factor 1 (TTF-1) are performed since positivity for TTF-1 is a criterion contributing to adenocarcinoma classification.

  - Limitations of molecular techniques for tissue analysis are related to the choice of antibody as well as the choice of detection, scoring systems and cutoffs. These probably contribute to varied results reported in studies that test for EGFR expression.
  - Although IHC, FISH, and mutational assay techniques can be performed on cytology specimens, the absence of histologic architecture in cytology samples complicates the interpretation of IHC and FISH assay results, which require measure of the percentage or number of tumor cells that are positive.
- Almost 70 % of patients with lung cancer today are diagnosed based on small biopsies or cytology specimens (37). In these cases, adequate tissue samples may not be available for analysis by IHC, FISH or other ancillary studies requiring formalin-fixed, paraffin embedded (FFPE) tissue.
  - Optimizing FISH analysis and mutational analysis also depends on proper sample handling, preparation, and analysis (38).
  - Although IHC and FISH can be technically applied to NSCLC cytology specimens such as FNA cytospin cell blocks, the approaches to interpreting the assays are not yet established and validated (38);
  - For EFGR FISH and IHC analysis, it is currently recommended that a tumor tissue section should contain at least 1 to 2mm^2 of tumor area to provide enough tumor cells for reliable interpretation. FISH results should include hybridization signal counts from at least 100 to 200 tumor cells that meet the morphologic and quality criteria for being acceptable for evaluation (38).
  - For mutational analysis, larger amounts of tissue might be required to ensure that sufficient DNA is obtained (38).
  - The type of analysis, once a firm pathologic diagnosis is obtained, is impacted by the choice of tissue sample and the method of preservation (39).
  - Standardized protocols for specimen collection and handling are needed to improve the reproducibility and consistency of molecular analyses.

- **Handling EBUS-TBNA specimens**: The following steps have been proposed for handling EBUS-TBNA specimens destined for possible molecular analysis (40). (*Note from the authors: This can be addressed as part of a hands-on workstation).See Tissue Sampling video (Bronch.org site on YouTube).
  1. The aspirated material is pushed out onto the glass slide with the inner stylet.
  2. The tissue core (if obtained) is placed on filter paper in order to absorb excess blood:
     a. Histopathologic samples obtained by core-needle biopsy or surgical resection are most commonly used to ensure adequate tissue for molecular testing in patients with NSCLC. Preliminary data indicate no significant difference in mutation rates between samples obtained by cytology versus histology (21). Several studies describe using routinely collected cytology specimens, such as smears or cell blocks, for molecular testing in patients with NSCLC (41-44).
     b. The core tissue is fixed with 10% neutral buffered formalin and a formalin-fixed paraffin-embedded (FFPE) sample is made. This is later stained with hematoxylin and eosin for histologic diagnosis and IHC. This specimen can also be used for FISH and for DNA/

RNA extraction for mutation assays. Formalin-fixed samples are preferred for histologic classification and some molecular assays (38), but fixation times have not been standardized. Following paraffin embedding, samples should be stored as a block to maintain the integrity of the antigens being analyzed.

   c. Part of the core can be stored (- 80 degree Celsius) using stabilizing solutions for RNA extraction.

3. The rest of the aspirated material is smeared onto glass slides[7] for:
   a. Air dried smears: stained by Diff-Quick or Giemsa stain solution for rapid on-site examination (45); for cytology specimens, an onsite pathologist can determine whether tissue samples are adequate depending on intended downstream analysis[8];
   b. 95% ethanol fixed smears: Papanicolau staining (45) is performed after checking the quality of the specimen's cellularity microscopically.
4. The needle is then rinsed into a tube with normal saline for
   a. Cell block.
   b. Flow cytometry, if indicated by clinical suspicion and differential diagnosis.
   c. Microbiology if indicated by clinical suspicion and differential diagnosis.
   d. DNA/RNA extraction.

Molecular Analysis-based Strategies for NSCLC Using EBUS-TBNA Samples

- Some oncologists apply testing and treatment algorithms when they encounter any new patient with advanced NSCLC (1).
  - First, EGFR mutation analysis: if there is a mutation, the patient is a candidate for EGFR-TKI (18).
  - If there is no response, or if the mutation is not present, than the tumor is assessed for EML4/ALK rearrangements and if present, treated with crizotinib (30).
  - Second, if there is no response or evidence of EML4/ALK fusion, then the tumor is assessed for ERCC1 and RRM 1. Patients with low levels are treated with platinum plus gemcitabine combination (46). If there is no response, the levels of ERCC1 and TS are assessed. Patients with low ERCC1 and TS levels are treated with a platinum plus pemetrexed combination.
  - For patients who fail these treatments or who have high levels of ERCC1, default treatment is with a taxane plus a non-platinum drug.
- Non-Small Cell Lung Cancer NCCN Guidelines recommend that molecular diagnostic studies be included in the pathologic evaluation of NSCLC (www.nccn.org).
  - Histologic type should be established before EGRF testing.
  - EGFR mutation testing should be performed on adenocarcinoma, large cell carcinoma, and NSCLC not otherwise specified.

---

[7] Specimen adequacy for smears and cell-block preparations were comparable when analyzed for EGFR and KRAS mutation by direct sequencing.

[8] Therefore, the bronchoscopist needs to balance these concerns against a need to minimize patient discomfort and procedural complications if choosing to obtain larger tumor samples.

  - Testing for EGFR is not recommended for squamous cell carcinoma, which has a mutation rate of ~3.6%.
  - KRAS mutations are associated with intrinsic TKI resistance, and KRAS testing could be used for the selection of patients as candidates for TKI therapy.
  - EGFR mutations are generally exclusive of ALK rearrangements.ALK testing should not be considered for those who test positive for EGFR mutation.
  - Patients with advanced NSCLC who progressed on previous therapy and have the EML4-ALK oncogene benefit from EML4-ALK inhibitors such as crizotinib.
- For practical purposes, bronchoscopists may want to perform more than the three to four aspirates usually considered necessary for tissue diagnosis. Ideally core biopsies are obtained so that specimens can be preserved for further molecular analysis. As of this writing, prioritization of specimens for molecular analysis is considered after specimens are first obtained for accurate diagnosis and staging.
- In this era of individualized care and because the majority of patients with advanced NSCLC are diagnosed using small volume specimens, there is a need for continued development of assay technologies to optimize the usefulness of smaller samples (38).
- Multidisciplinary NSCLC working groups including oncologists, pathologists, chest physicians, thoracic surgeons and scientists with special expertise in the clinical applications of molecular biology are warranted to help determine which molecular assays are most applicable to EBUS- TBNA specimens as well as establish uniform standardized methods of processing[9].

References

1. Gadgeel SM, Cote ML, Schwartz AG, et al. Parameters for individualizing systemic therapy in non-small cell lung cancer. Drug Resist Updat 2010;13:196-204.
2. Gazdar AF. Tyrosine kinase inhibitors and epidermal growth factor receptor (EGFR) mutations in non-small cell lung cancer: to test or not to test? Medicine 2011; 90: 168-170.
3. Brose MS, Volpe P, Feldman M, et al. BRAF and RAS mutations in lung cancer and melanoma. Cancer Res 62:6997-7000, 2002.
4. Schmid K, Oehl N, Wiba F, et al. EGFR/KRAS/BRAF mutations in primary lung adenocarcinomas and corresponding locoregional lymph node metastases. Clin Cancer Res 2009;15:4554-4560.
5. Koivunen JP, Mermel C, Zejnullahu K, et al. EML4-ALK fusion gene and efficacy of an ALK kinase inhibitor in lung cancer. Clin Cancer Res 2008;14:4275-4283.
6. Martelli MP, Sozzi G, Hernandez L, et al. EML4-ALK rearrangement in non-small cell lung cancer and non-tumor lung tissues. Am J Pathol 2009;174:661-670.
7. Printz C. BATTLE to personalize lung cancer treatment. Novel clinical trial design and tissue gathering procedures drive biomarker discovery. Cancer. 2010;116:3307-8.
8. Reed E. ERCC1 and clinical resistance to platinum-based therapy. Clin Cancer Res 2005; 11:6100-6102.

[9] In this regard, as far as EGFR is concerned, it is currently recommended that all pathology reports include an accurate description of the sample type (eg, solid tissue block of tumor resection, excisional biopsy, endobronchial biopsy, or core needle biopsy; cytospin cell block; or cytology smears), fixative and fixation conditions, whether an enrichment technique such as microdissection was used, and the approximate number of tumor cells (eg,< 100, 100 to 1,000,>1,000 cells) or tumor section area (in micrometers squared or mm2) included in the assay performance or interpretation (38).

9. Simon GR, Sharma S, Cantor A, et al. ERCC1 expression is a predictor of survival in resected patients with non-small cell lung cancer. Chest 2005; 127: 978-983.
10. Olaussen KA, Dunant A, Fouret P, et al. DNA repair by ERCC1 in non-small-cell lung cancer and cisplatin-based adjuvant chemotherapy. N Engl J Med. 2006;355:983-991.
11. Bepler G, Sharma S, Cantor A, et al. RRM1 and PTEN as prognostic parameters for overall and disease-free survival in patients with nonsmall- cell lung cancer. J Clin Oncol. 2004;22:1878-1885.
12. Rosell R, Danenberg KD, Alberola V, et al; Spanish Lung Cancer Group. Ribonucleotide reductase messenger RNA expression and survival in gemcitabine/cisplatin-treated advanced non-small cell lung cancer patients. Clin Cancer Res 2004; 10:1318-1325.
13. Bepler G, Kusmartseva I, Sharma S, et al. RRM1modulated in vitro and in vivo efficacy of gemcitabine and platinum in non-small-cell lung cancer. J Clin Oncol 2006; 24:4731-4737.
14. West H, Lilenbaum R, Harpole D, et al. Molecular analysis-based treatment strategies for the management of non-small cell lung cancer. J Thorac Oncol. 2009;4 (9 Suppl 2):S1029-39.
15. Scagliotti GV, Parikh P, von Pawel J, et al. Phase III study comparing cisplatin plus gemcitabine with cisplatin plus pemetrexed in chemotherapy-naive patients with advanced-stage non-small-cell lung cancer. J Clin Oncol 2008; 26:3543-3551.
16. Maemondo M, Inoue A, Kobayashi K, et al. Gefitinib or chemotherapy for non-small-cell lung cancer with mutated EGFR. N Engl J Med 2010; 362: 2380-2388.
17. Shih JY, Gow CH, Yu CJ, et al. Epidermal growth factor receptor mutations in needle biopsy/aspiration samples predict response to gefitinib therapy and survival of patients with advanced nonsmall cell lung cancer. Int. J. Cancer 2006: 118; 963–969.
18. Mok TS, Wu YL, Thongprasert S, et al: Gefitinib or carboplatin-paclitaxel in pulmonary adenocarcinoma. N Engl J Med 2009; 361:947-957.
19. John T, Liu G, Tsao MS. Overview of molecular testing in non-small-cell lung cancer: mutational analysis, gene copy number, protein expression and other biomarkers of EGFR for the prediction of response to tyrosine kinase inhibitors. Oncogene. 2009;28 suppl 1:S14-S23.
20. D'Cunha J. "Personalizing" therapy for non-small cell lung cancer. Semin Thorac Cardiovasc Surg. 2010;22(2):118-20.
21. Billah S, Stewart J, Staerkel G, et al. EGFR and KRAS mutations in lung carcinoma: molecular testing by using cytology specimens. Cancer (Cancer Cytopathol) 2011; 119: 111–7.
22. Penzel R, Sers C, Chen Y, et al. EGFR mutation detection in NSCLC--assessment of diagnostic application and recommendations of the German Panel for Mutation Testing in NSCLC. Virchows Arch. 2011;458:95-8.
23. Nakajima T, Yasufuku K, Nakagawara A, et al. Multi-gene mutation analysis of metastatic lymph nodes in non-small cell lung cancer diagnosed by EBUS-TBNA. Chest. 2011 Apr 28 [Epub ahead of print].
24. Nakajima T, Yasufuku K, Suzuki M, et al. Assessment of epidermal growth factor receptor mutation by endobronchial ultrasound-guided transbronchial needle aspiration. Chest. 2007; 132: 597-602.
25. Garcia-Olivé I, Monsó E, Andreo F et al. Endobronchial ultrasound-guided transbronchial needle aspiration for identifying EGFR mutations. Eur Respir J. 2010; 35: 391-5.
26. Hammerman PS, Janne PA, Johnson BE. Resistance to epidermal growth factor receptor tyrosine kinase inhibitors in non small cell lung cancer. Clin Cancer Res. 2009;15:7502-7509.
27. Eberhard DA, Johnson BE, Amler LC, et al. Mutations in the epidermal growth factor receptor and in KRAS are predictive and prognostic indicators in patients with non-small-cell lung cancer treated with chemotherapy alone and in combination with erlotinib. J Clin Oncol. 2005;23:5900-5909.
28. Mohamed S, Yasufuku K, Nakajima T. Analysis of cell cycle-related proteins in mediastinal lymph nodes of patients with N2-NSCLC obtained by EBUS-TBNA: relevance to chemotherapy response. Thorax. 2008; 63: 642-7.
29. Solomon B, Varella-Garcia M, Camidge DR. ALK gene rearrangements: a new therapeutic target in a molecularly defined subset of non-small cell lung cancer. J Thorac Oncol. 2009; 4: 1450-1454.
30. Kwak EL, Bang YJ, Camidge DR, et al: Anaplastic lymphoma kinase inhibition in non-small-cell lung cancer. N Engl J Med 2010; 363:1693-1703.

31. Ou SH, Bazhenova L, Camidge DR, et al. Rapid and dramatic radiographic and clinical response to an ALK inhibitor (crizotinib, PF02341066) in an ALK translocation-positive patient with non-small cell lung cancer. J Thorac Oncol 2010; 5:2044-2046.
32. Sakairi Y, Nakajima T, Yasufuku K, et al. EML4-ALK fusion gene assessment using metastatic lymph node samples obtained by endobronchial ultrasound-guided transbronchial needle aspiration. Clin Cancer Res. 2010;16:4938-45.
33. Bunn PA Jr, Doebele RC. Genetic testing for lung cancer: reflex versus clinical selection. J Clin Oncol. 2011;29:1943-5.
34. Paik PK, Arcila ME, Fara M, et al. Clinical characteristics of patients with lung adenocarcinomas harboring *BRAF* mutations. J Clin Oncol 2011; 29:2046-2059.
35. Schmid K, Oehl N, Wrba F, et al. EGFR/KRAS/BRAF mutations in primary lung adenocarcinomas and corresponding locoregional lymph node metastases. Clin Cancer Res 2009;15:4554-4560.
36. Potti A, Mukherjee S, Petersen R, et al. A genomic strategy to refine prognosis in early-stage non-small-cell lung cancer. N Engl J Med. 2006;355:570-80.
37. Travis WD, Brambilla E, Noguchi M, et al. International association for the study of lung cancer/american thoracic society/european respiratory society international multidisciplinary classification of lung adenocarcinoma. *J Thorac Oncol.* 2011:6:244-85.
38. Eberhard DA, Giaccone G, Johnson BE. Biomarkers of response to epidermal growth factor receptor inhibitors in Non- Small-Cell Lung Cancer Working Group: standardization for use in the clinical trial setting. J Clin Oncol 2008; 26:983–994
39. West H, Harpole D, Travis W. Histologic considerations for individualized systemic therapy approaches for the management of non-small cell lung cancer. Chest 2009; 136:1112–1118.
40. Nakajima T, Yasufuku K. How I do it--optimal methodology for multidirectional analysis of endobronchial ultrasound-guided transbronchial needle aspiration samples. J Thorac Oncol. 2011;6:203-6.
41. Wu SG, Gow CH, Yu CJ, et al. Frequent epidermal growth factor receptor gene mutations in malignant pleural effusion of lung adenocarcinoma. Eur Respir J. 2008;32:924-930.
42. Smouse JH, Cibas ES, Janne PA, et al. EGFR mutations are detected comparably in cytologic and surgical pathology specimens of nonsmall cell lung cancer. Cancer Cytopathol. 2009;117:67-72.
43. Smith GD, Chadwick BE, Willmore-Payne C, et al. Detection of epidermal growth factor receptor gene mutations in cytology specimens from patients with non-small cell lung cancer utilizing high-resolution melting amplicon analysis. J Clin Pathol. 2008;61:487-493.
44. Nomoto K, Tsuta K, Takano T, et al. Detection of EGFR mutations in archived cytologic specimens of non-small cell lung cancer using high-resolution melting analysis. Am J Clin Pathol. 2006;126: 608-615.
45. Cameron SE, Andrade RS, Pambuccian SE. Endobronchial ultrasound-guided transbronchial needle aspiration cytology: a state of the art review. Cytopathology 2010; 21:6-26.
46. Reynolds C, Obasaju C, Schell MJ, et al. Randomized phase III trial of gemcitabine-based chemotherapy with in situ RRM1 and ERCC1 protein levels for response prediction in non-small-cell lung cancer. J Clin Oncol 2009; 27:5808-15.

Glossary of Key Terms Used in this Synopsis

- *DNA(Deoxyribonucleic acid):* a nucleic acid that consists of two long chains of nucleotides twisted together into a double helix and joined by hydrogen bonds between complementary bases adenine and thymine or cytosine and guanine. DNA carries the cell's genetic information and hereditary characteristics via its nucleotides and their sequence. DNA is capable of self-replication and RNA synthesis (http://medical-dictionary.thefreedictionary.com/DNA; accessed 8/6/2011).

- *DNA damage repair:* a series of enzymatic mechanisms whereby errors or damage to one of the two DNA strands are removed by excision and replaced by correct nucleotides using the undamaged strand as a template. (http://medical-dictionary.thefreedictionary.com/DNA+repair; accessed 8/6/2011).
- *DNA sequencing:* a method in which DNA is synthesized in vitro in such a way that it is radioactively labeled. The reaction terminates specifically at the position corresponding to a given base.
- *EGFR (*Epidermal Growth Factor Receptor): a cell adhesion process protein encoded by the human EGFR gene. EGFR has roles in cell-cell adhesion, cell migration, cell proliferation and signal transduction (http://de.dict.md/definition/EGF; accessed 8/6/2011).
- *EGFR signaling:* the series of molecular signals generated as a consequence of an epidermal growth factor receptor binding to one of its physiological ligands (http://de.dict.md/definition/EGF; accessed 8/6/2011).
- *Exons*: portion of a gene included in the transcript of a gene that survives processing of the RNA in the cell nucleus to become part of a spliced messenger of structural RNA in the cell cytoplasm; an exon specifies the amino acid sequence of a portion of the complete polypeptide. http://www.kumc.edu/gec/glossnew.html; accessed 8/6/2011).
- *Fluorescence in situ hybridization* (*FISH):* a technique for uniquely identifying whole chromosomes or parts of chromosomes using florescent tagged DNA.
- *Gene:* according to the official Guidelines for Human Gene Nomenclature, a gene is defined as a DNA segment that contributes to phenotype/function (http://www.genenames.org/guidelines.html; accessed 8/6/2011).
- *Gene expression:* Process by which information from a gene is used in the synthesis of a functional gene product (either RNA or protein).
- *Gene over-expression (high expression):* excessive expression of a gene by producing too much of its effect or product.
- *Gene fusion:* the genetic recombination of the parts of two or more genes resulting in a gene with different or additional regulatory regions, or a new chimeric gene product; oncogene fusion includes an oncogene as at least one of the fusion partners. Such gene fusions are often detected in neoplastic cells and are transcribed into oncogene fusion proteins (http://www.definitions.net/definition/gene%20fusion; accessed 8/6/2011).
- *Genome:* all of the genes carried by a single gamete. This provides the DNA content of an individual, which includes all 44 autosomes, 2 sex chromosomes, and mitochondrial DNA.
- *Genotype:* genetic constitution of an organism.
- *High resolution melt analysis (HRMAA):* molecular biology technique used for the detection of mutations in double-stranded DNA samples.
- *Mutation:* process by which genes undergo a structural change.
- *Messenger RNA (mRNA):* RNA molecules, usually 400 to 10,000 bases long, that serve as templates for protein synthesis (translation) (http://medical-dictionary.thefreedictionary.com/RNA; accessed 8/6/2011).
- *Nucleotides:* molecules that, when joined together, make up the structural units of RNA and DNA.
- *Nucleotide metabolism:* sum of chemical changes that occur within the tissues of an organism consisting of anabolism (biosynthesis) and catabolism of nucleotides; the buildup and breakdown

of nucleotides for utilization by the organism (http://de.dict.md/definition/nucleotides; accessed 8/6/2011).

- *Oligonucleotide:* a short piece of nucleic acid, usually with less than twenty nucleotides, used in genetic engineering and research.
- *Oncogenic driver mutation:* "A driver mutation is causally implicated in oncogenesis. It has conferred growth advantage on the cancer cell and has been positively selected in the microenvironment of the tissue in which the cancer arises ("The cancer genome. Michael R. Stratton, Peter J. Campbell & P. Andrew Futreal *Nature* **458**, 719-724(9 April 2009) doi:10.1038/nature07943).
- *Oncogene:* genes involved in cell cycle control (growth factors, growth factor regulator genes, etc). A mutation can lead to tumor growth.
- *PCR (polymerase chain reaction):* a technique for rapidly producing many copies of a fragment of DNA for diagnostic or research purposes.
- *Phenotype:* the complete observable characteristics of an organism or group, including anatomic, physiologic, biochemical, and behavioral traits as determined by the interaction of genetic makeup and environmental factors (http://medical-dictionary.thefreedictionary.com; accessed 8/6/2011).
- *RNA (ribonucleic acid):* a polymeric constituent of all living cells and many viruses. Consists of a long, usually single-stranded chain of alternating phosphate and ribose units with the bases adenine, guanine, cytosine, and uracil bonded to the ribose. The structure and base sequence of RNA are determinants of protein synthesis and the transmission of genetic information. (http://medical-dictionary.thefreedictionary.com/RNA; accessed 8/6/2011).
- *RT-PCR (Reverse transcription polymerase chain reaction):* is a variant of polymerase chain reaction (PCR), a technique used to generate many copies of a DNA sequence (amplification).
- *Tyrosine kinase (TK):* an enzyme intimately linked to signal transduction, either as a receptor-type TK, which participates in transmembrane signaling, or as an intracellular TK, participating in signal transduction to the nucleus (http://medical-dictionary.thefreedictionary.com/tyrosine+kinase; accessed 8/6/2011).
- *Tyrosine kinase inhibitor (TKI):* a drug that inhibits tyrosine kinases.

Clinical Pathway: EBUS-TBNA and Molecular Analysis in Advanced NSCLC

The purpose of this example of a clinical pathway exercise is to provide an opportunity for the reader to apply cognitive knowledge to a patient-centered case scenario. The reader should respond to each of the multiple choice questions prior to reading the answer. Each answer addresses each of the multiple choice responses, and provides material that is complementary to other learning materials providing in this training manual. Pertinent references are provided after each question.

Case Description: A 65 year old Spanish woman with no history of smoking saw her primary care physician for preoperative medical clearance before knee surgery. A chest radiograph showed a 4 X 5 cm mass in the right upper lobe. Computed tomography confirmed the mass and also showed a 1.2 cm right lower paratracheal lymph node, a 1 cm left lower paratracheal node, and a 1.7 cm subcarinal node. Whole body PET CT was then performed, which showed increased uptake in the primary tumor and in the three mediastinal lymph nodes. Brain MRI was negative.

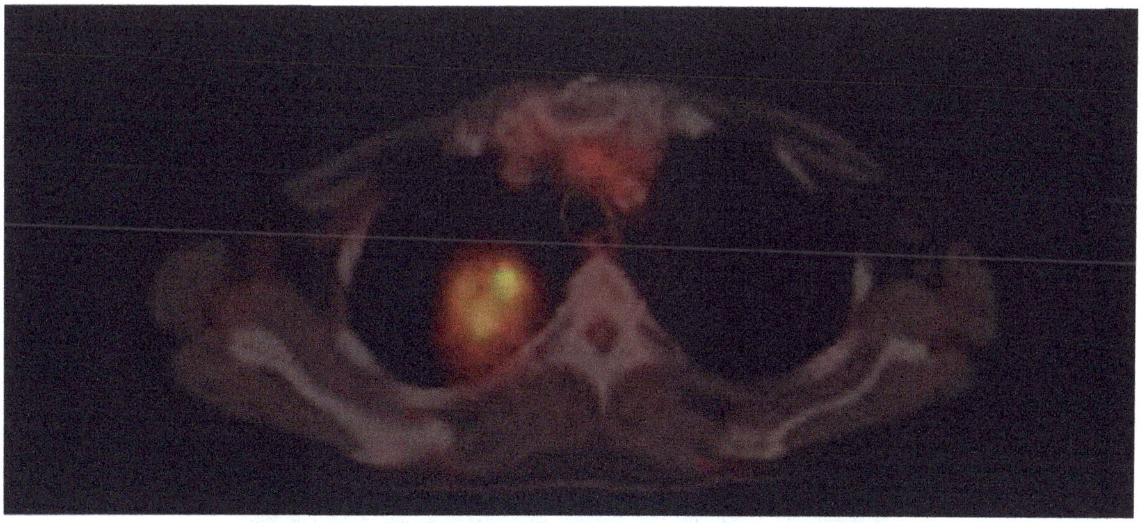

Question 1: Which of the following three procedures are now indicated? Please justify your choice.

A. Mediastinoscopy
B. EBUS-guided TBNA
C. Conventional TBNA

Response: B. Any of the three procedures could be performed and could make the diagnosis. For lymph node station 4L, however, the yield is higher with EBUS-TBNA than with conventional TBNA[1]. Mediastinoscopy provides systematic exploration and biopsy under visual guidance of nodal stations 1, 2, 3, 4 and 7 but has associated morbidity. Diagnosis can probably be obtained bronchoscopically (stations 4R, 4L, and 7) or endoscopically (stations 4L and 7). Data from a meta-analysis of EBUS-TBNA for patients with confirmed or suspected NSCLC showed that a subgroup of patients selected on the basis of CT or PET positive results had a pooled sensitivity of 94%, higher than a subgroup of patients who had not been selected according to CT or PET results (sensitivity 76%) [2]. The patient in this case has an enlarged, PET positive lymph node. The yield of EBUS-TBNA is expected to be greater than 90%. A negative EBUS-TBNA in patients with highly suspected mediastinal nodal involvement, however, should be followed by mediastinoscopy. In fact, up to 28% of patients with a high clinical suspicion of nodal disease could have mediastinal nodal metastases confirmed by mediastinoscopy despite negative EBUS-TBNA[3].

References:

1. Herth FJ, Lunn W, Eberhardt R, et al. Transbronchial versus transesophageal ultrasound-guided aspiration of enlarged mediastinal lymph nodes. Am J Respir Crit Care Med. 2005 May 15;171:1164-7.
2. Gu P, Zhao Y, Jiang L, et al. Endobronchial ultrasound-guided transbronchial needle aspiration for staging of lung cancer: A systematic review and meta-analysis. Eur J Cancer 2009; 45, 1389-1396.
3. Defranchi SA, Edell ES, Daniels C E et al. Mediastinoscopy in Patients with Lung Cancer and Negative Endobronchial Ultrasound Guided Needle Aspiration. Ann Thorac Surg 2010; 90: 1753-8.

Case Continues: White light bronchoscopy and EBUS-TBNA were performed under general anesthesia and with rapid on site evaluation. No airway abnormalities were seen. EBUS examination of the mediastinum confirmed enlarged nodes at levels 4R, 4L and 7, and revealed no other mediastinal or hilar abnormalities.

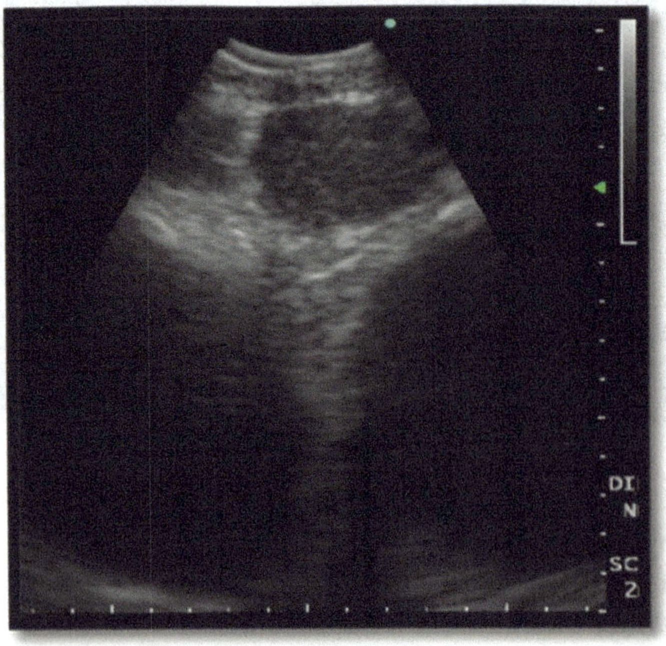

Question 2: Which lymph node station should be sampled first? Please justify your response.

A. Station 4R
B. Station 4L
C. Station 7

Response: **B**. Overall, diagnostic yield from conventional TBNA and EBUS-TBNA is highest from subcarinal nodes (station 7). This argues for initially sampling the subcarinal node in this patient. The first station that should be sampled, however, is station 4L because the patient has a right upper lobe mass, and a station 4L contra-lateral mediastinal node (N3), in addition to N2 nodes at stations 7 and 4R[1]. If N3 nodes are positive for malignancy on rapid on-site cytological evaluation (ROSE), and if the goal is diagnosis and mediastinal staging only (i.e. stage III B, in this example), the procedure could be terminated. Should the contralateral node be negative, than either station 4R or 7 could be sampled, and of positive, the patient will have stage III A disease.

References:

1. Herth F, Lunn W, Eberhardt R, et al. Transbronchial versus transesophageal ultrasound guided needle aspiration of enlarged mediastinal lymph nodes. Eur Respir J 2006; 28: 910-914

Case Continues: A first aspirate was done from the level 4L node. Rapid on-site examination was positive for malignancy, favoring adenocarcinoma. Using a 22 gauge needle the second aspirate showed core tissue. Part of the core was placed in formalin for histopathology and part was placed in stabilizing solution to be later used for DNA and RNA extraction.

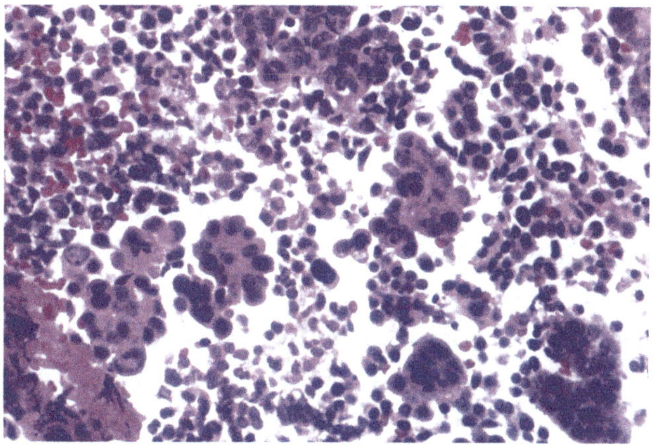

Question 3: At this point you choose to:

A. Terminate the procedure
B. Perform at least two more aspirates from the level 4L node
C. Obtain additional aspirations from the level 7 and level 4R node.

Response: B. All choices are potentially correct. Bronchoscopists should communicate with the Pathology department in their institutions to determine a level of confidence for diagnosing lung carcinoma on rapid on-site evaluation (ROSE). In general, there is a good correlation between ROSE and the final cytologic diagnosis, so aborting the procedure could be the appropriate next step. In this case, after specimen adequacy is established and the diagnosis of malignancy is made, the patient is classified as having N3 disease (stage III B); therefore, the procedure could be terminated after the first two aspirates. Indeed, evidence suggests that optimal results are obtained after three aspirations per lymph node station and that when at least one tissue-core specimen is obtained by the first or second aspiration, two aspirations per station are acceptable[1].

Obtaining at least two additional aspirates from station 4L is desirable in this patient, however, because adequate specimen is needed for molecular analysis. If this patient's diagnosis is confirmed to be adenocarcinoma as suspected by ROSE, targeted therapy might be considered either as a first or second line treatment for locally advanced disease; this depends, however, on the biomarker analysis, for which adequate specimens are needed. For instance, specimens are considered adequate for EGFR analysis if they contain more than 40% malignant cells which could be obtained by four "good" fine needle aspirations or 2-3 core needle tissues[2].

Sampling station 7 and 4R is also possible if more tissue is needed for downstream molecular analysis but is not necessary for staging. ROSE will be necessary to confirm the presence of malignant cells and the adequate cellularity necessary before submitting the specimen to the molecular pathology laboratory. This can increase the time and cost of the procedure, and potentially compromise patient safety because of prolonged procedure. Sending the specimen directly for molecular analysis without confirming the presence of malignancy first may not be cost effective because biopsy specimens may contain limited amount of carcinoma cells sufficient for molecular testing[3].

References:

1. Lee HS, Lee GK, Lee HS, et al. Real-time endobronchial ultrasound-guided transbronchial needle aspiration in mediastinal staging of non-small cell lung cancer: how many aspirations per target lymph node station? Chest. 2008;134:368-74.
2. http://labmed.ucsf.edu/uploads/369/166_24JonesMolecularPathologyOfLungCancer.pdf (accessed 8/23/11).
3. Coghlin CL, Smith LJ, Bakar S, et al. Quantitative analysis of tumor in bronchial biopsy specimens. J Thorac Oncol. 2010;5:448-52.

Case Continues: After obtaining two more aspirates from level 4L, you decide to obtain additional aspirates from level 7. The first aspirate at this level is positive for malignancy, most likely adenocarcinoma. You obtain three additional samples to send to the laboratory for biomarkers.

Question 4: You choose to submit these samples for which of the following tests?

A. EGFR (mutation analysis)
B. KRAS (mutation analysis)
C. EML4-ALK gene rearrangement by FISH

Response: A. Results from all three tests can alter patient management. EGFR (epidermal growth factor receptor) is a growth promoting protein lying within the cytoplasmic membrane; its external domain binds growth factors and is the target of large monoclonal antibody drugs such as cetuximab while the internal domain, including the tyrosine kinase domain, is the target of small molecule drugs, known as tyrosine kinase inhibitors (TKIs). EGFR mutation positivity will predict response to TKIs. Phenotypically, this patient has increased risk for having an EGFR mutation: female, non- smoker and with adenocarcinoma[1]. One characteristic that may not be an increased factor is her Caucasian race; however, EGFR mutations are seen in approximately 10 -20 % of Caucasians and recent data suggest these patients, similar to East Asian patients, benefit from TKIs in terms of response rate and progression free survival[2].

Fine needle aspirates, unstained slides and formalin fixed paraffin embedded (FFPE) tissues, when core tissue is obtained, can be sent for EGFR mutation analysis (by RT-PCR technique), protein over-expression (by immunohistochemistry) or increased gene copy number (by fluorescent in situ hybridization)[3]. Relevant to this patient, EGFR mutation analysis is feasible in needle biopsy/aspiration paraffin-fixed specimens such as EBUS-TBNA. EGFR mutation has been reported in 10-37% of EBUS-TBNA specimens. In one study using a PCR technique, the overall specimen insufficiency rate for EBUS was only 4%, a rate that is lower than by CT guided biopsy[4].

KRAS mutation occurs in approximately 15-30% of NSCLC, mostly in lung adenocarcinoma, rarely in squamous cell carcinoma and is mutually exclusive with EGFR mutations. This mutation is associated with smoking history, male gender, western population, with poor prognosis and rapid disease progression; its presence confers resistance to treatment with TKIs. These mutations were detected by DNA sequencing in 3.5-7% of EBUS-TBNA specimens, but the optimal methodology for the detection of KRAS mutation for needle biopsied samples is uncertain at this time; in fact, needle specimens may be inadequate since resected specimens show the mutation at higher frequencies[4].

The anaplastic lymphoma kinase (ALK) is a receptor tyrosine kinase that is aberrant in a variety of malignancies. The EML4-ALK fusion oncogene results from a small inversion within chromosome 2p. This leads to expression of a chimeric tyrosine kinase, in which the N-terminal half of echinoderm microtubule-associated protein-like 4 (EML4) is fused to the intracellular kinase domain of ALK. Approximately 3-7% of lung tumors harbor ALK fusions and in the vast majority of cases, ALK rearrangements are non-overlapping with other oncogenic mutations found in NSCLC (i.e. EGFR mutations, KRAS mutations). Clinically, the presence of EML4-ALK fusions is associated with EGFR TKI resistance[3]. ALK gene rearrangement is usually tested for by fluorescence in situ hybridization (FISH) and require at least 2 mL of special media for fine needle aspirates or 10% neutral buffered FFPE tissue; it can also be detected by immunohistochemistry and RT-PCR and is feasible in EBUS-TBNA specimens[5]. EML4-ALK gene rearrangement predicts response to crizotinib, an inhibitor of the chimeric tyrosine kinase synthesized by this oncogene and could therefore assist in the management of this patient.

References:

1. Rosell R, Moran T, Queralt C, et al; Spanish Lung Cancer Group. Screening for epidermal growth factor receptor mutations in lung cancer. N Engl J Med. 2009;361:958-67
2. R. Rosell, R. Gervais, A. Vergnenegre, et al. Erlotinib versus chemotherapy (CT) in advanced non-small cell lung cancer (NSCLC) patients (p) with epidermal growth factor receptor (EGFR) mutations: Interim results of the European Erlotinib Versus Chemotherapy (EURTAC) phase III randomized trial. J Clin Oncol 29: 2011 (suppl; abstr 7503)
3. http://www.mycancergenome.org/molecular-pathology (accessed 8/23/11)

4. Nakajima T, Yasufuku K, Nakagawara A, et al. Multi-gene mutation analysis of metastatic lymph nodes in non-small cell lung cancer diagnosed by EBUS-TBNA. Chest 2011 Apr 28. [Epub ahead of print]
5. Sakairi Y, Nakajima T, Yasufuku K, et al. EML4-ALK fusion gene assessment using metastatic lymph node samples obtained by endobronchial ultrasound-guided transbronchial needle aspiration. Clin Cancer Res. 2010;16:4938-45.

Case Continues: After obtaining all the specimens, the procedure is terminated, and the patient is transferred to the recovery area and discharged home. On follow-up visit, the final results of the procedure are discussed. The patient has primary lung adenocarcinoma, EGFR mutation analysis showed deletion of exon 19; KRAS mutation was negative and EML4-ALK rearrangement was negative by FISH.

Question 5: As of this writing, this patient will most likely benefit from which of the following?

A. crizotinib
B. erlotinib
C. pemetrexed

Response: B. The oncogenic activity of the chimeric tyrosine kinase resulting from expression of EML4-ALK fusion oncogene can be effectively blocked by small molecular inhibitors such as crizotinib.

Evidence suggest that patients with advanced NSCLC whose tumors harbor EML4-ALK fusion genes and who are treated with the ALK TKI crizotinib have high response rates and long progression-free survival times similar to those of patients with NSCLC and EGFR mutations who are treated with erlotinib[1].

Erlotinib and geftinib are EGFR TKIs that increase the response rate and progression free survival compared with chemotherapy. This effect was seen in patients who were mutation positive and received TKI, geftinib, compared with those who received carboplatin/paclitaxel[2]. The response rate in mutation positive patients was 73.7% versus 30.7 % and progression free survival (PFS) was 10.8 versus 5.4 months favoring geftinib[3]. Similar response rates are seen in the Caucasian population with 58% objective response for erlotinib compared with 15% for chemotherapy; improved progression free survival from 5.2 months to 9.4 months[4]. Pemetrexed is a drug used in NSCLC in patients with a low level of thymidylate synthase (TS) expression. This enzyme involved in DNA biosynthesis is responsible for maintaining intracellular levels of thymidine, important for DNA synthesis and repair. Immunohistochemistry and RT-PCR on FFPE tissue can be analyzed for TS expression (mRNA) which is higher in patients with squamous cell carcinoma compared to adenocarcinoma and is correlated with resistance to pemetrexed[5].

References:

1. Kwak EL, Bang YJ, Camidge DR, et al. Anaplastic lymphoma kinase inhibition in non-small-cell lung cancer. N Engl J Med 2010; 363:1693-1703.
2. Mok TS, Wu YL, Thongprasert S, et al. Gefitinib or carboplatin-paclitaxel in pulmonary adenocarcinoma. N Engl J Med. 2009;361: 947-57.
3. Maemondo M, Inoue A, Kobayashi K, et al; North-East Japan Study Group. Gefitinib or chemotherapy for non-small-cell lung cancer with mutated EGFR. N Engl J Med. 2010;362:2380-8.

4. R. Rosell, R. Gervais, A. Vergnenegre, et al. Erlotinib versus chemotherapy (CT) in advanced non-small cell lung cancer (NSCLC) patients (p) with epidermal growth factor receptor (EGFR) mutations: Interim results of the European Erlotinib Versus Chemotherapy (EURTAC) phase III randomized trial. J Clin Oncol 29: 2011 (suppl; abstr 7503).
5. Scagliotti GV, Parikh P, von Pawel J, et al. Phase III study comparing cisplatin plus gemcitabine with cisplatin plus pemetrexed in chemotherapy-naive patients with advanced-stage non-small-cell lung cancer. J Clin Oncol 2008; 26:3543-3551.

****

SECTION 4

EBUS Step-by-Step

The EBUS Bronchoscopy Step-by-Step presentation is based on the idea that with patience, each step can be mastered. To become a good tennis player, one cannot master the forehand, backhand, serve, volley, smash and all other strokes at the same time; separately and repeatedly, different strokes are practiced and then combined to play a beautiful game. The same holds true for the multiple steps needed to perform EBUS-TBNA. It is also necessary to communicate clearly to a bronchoscopy assistant who helps handle the needle and syringe, applies suction, and subsequently handles the specimen.

EBUS step by step therefore provides learners with a:

- *Systematic Approach:* Deconstructing a complex task into constituent elements
- *Development of Muscle Memory:* Motor learning through the sub-conscious process of improving motor skills, smoothness and accuracy of movements, thus creating maximum efficiency and economy of movement. The major prerequisite for development of muscle memory is *repeated, deliberate practice.*
- *Development of Spatial Awareness:* To learn to flow in space, always occupying the desired position. In EBUS bronchoscopy, this additionally requires the accurate identification of airway anatomy, manipulation of the 30 degree view EBUS scope, and appropriate positioning of the transducer within the airway.

EBUS Bronchoscopy Step-by-Step

The same principles as those applied to Flexible Bronchoscopy Step-by-Step are followed. Optimum hand position and posture should be maintained at all times. The bronchoscope's position within the airway should be known at all times, recalling that the angle of view is 30 degrees. The airway wall should be respected and trauma avoided during nodal sampling. Careful attention should be paid to the order in which lymph nodes are sampled. Contamination of needle entry sites or of the needle sheath and aspirating needle must be consistently avoided. Steps should be practiced while standing both at the "patient's" head and side, although it is most likely practitioners will be performing EBUS-TBNA from the head of the patient. It is best that practice be done initially on inanimate models and/or a virtual reality (VR) simulator.

Remember: Decision; Intent; Control; Confidence; Economy of Movement.

Background:

A curved array ultrasound transducer is built into the distal end of the EBUS bronchoscope which has a thirty degree field of vision using white light bronchoscopy. The processor has adjustable depth and gain. It also has Doppler capabilities to identify blood flow in vessels, distinguishing them from lymph nodes. The 22 gauge disposable needle and sheath protrude at an angle. The lockable sheath prevents injury to the scope during needle protrusion. An inner stylet prevents aspiration of bronchial cells.

Prior to EBUS, white light bronchoscopic inspection is performed and the airways are cleared of secretions. A touch control button on the ultrasound processor alternates between the bronchoscopic and ultrasound image. After airway inspection, the balloon can be inflated on the EBUS scope so that a small crescent of it is seen. It may be necessary to trouble shoot the balloon and needle/sheath apparatus (see Processor and Needle checklist as well as simulation scenarios). After sonographic mapping of the nodal and vascular structures of the mediastinum, the operator selects the target node(s) based on a predetermined strategy and proceeds with EBUS-TBNA. The following is just one example using a commercially available needle-syringe ensemble.

EBUS-TBNA in 15 steps (see EBUS step-by-step video)

1. The needle is inserted into the working channel.
2. The housing is secured to the bronchoscope by sliding the flange.

3. The sheath is released by twisting the inferior screw.
4. With the node visualized by US, the sheath is advanced out of the end of the scope until it slightly touches the airway wall. It is now safe to advance the needle.
5. The needle screw, located superiorly, is then released.
6. The needle is advanced by jabbing it into the lymph node.
7. During this process the needle may push the airway wall away from the balloon. The transducer –wall interface might become lost and the image may show reverberation artifact. This problem is overcome by gently advancing the scope or further inflating the balloon.
8. The needle is visualized within the lymph node.
9. The stylet is moved in and out a few times to dislodge bronchial epithelium or cellular debris that may have entered the needle.
10. The stylet is then withdrawn from the scope.
11. The syringe is attached to the needle and suction is applied.
12. The needle is moved back and forth within the node approximately 10 -15 times under ultrasound visualization.
13. Suction is released by removing the syringe from the scope.
14. The needle is retracted into the sheath.
15. The needle housing is unlocked and the needle and the sheath are removed together.

Disclaimer: The authors recognize that many needle-syringe ensembles are commercially available. Readers are encouraged to carefully review product inserts before performing EBUS-TBNA.

****

SECTION 5

Simulation Workshops

A series of *simulation workshops* that include:

- *EBUS Informed consent*, *Patient safety* and *Procedural pause.*
- *EBUS Airway access and Image acquisition* using inanimate models in order to demonstrate introduction of the EBUS bronchoscope through a laryngeal mask airway, endotracheal tube, and oral bite and the use of color Doppler, gain, depth, frequency and focus adjustments using the EBUS image processor
- *EBUS-TBNA needle and scope handling,* using inanimate models and/or high-fidelity computer-based simulation to practice needle handling and sampling of various lymph node stations.

* Checklists and assessment tools used at the discretion of program director.

USER INSTRUCTIONS

Simulation Workshops

The purpose of these workshops is for students to practice skills pertaining to EBUS and EBUS-TBNA without endangering or causing undue emotional or physical discomfort to patients. Using a combination of patient models, affordable low-fidelity case-based simulation, computer-based high-fidelity simulation, and interactive discussions and debriefing sessions, trainees and instructors work together to build a mutually productive educational environment consistent with the needs outlined in the ACGME Outcome Project.

Various assessment tools and *ten-point checklists* are used to document knowledge and skill acquisition in accordance with the elements required by ACGME (patient care, medical knowledge, practice-based learning and improvement, interpersonal communication skills, professionalism, and systems-based practice).

Case-based scenarios can be created by each training program, or scenarios already developed and tested can be used (some are downloadable from the Bronchoscopy.org website). Airway models, many of which are already being used internationally, can be purchased from organizations such as the American Association for Bronchology and Interventional Pulmonology and the Foundation for the Advancement of Medicine a (501-C3 nonprofit organization), as well as from private companies. Some can be loaned to institutions for specific courses.

Examples of Simulation Models

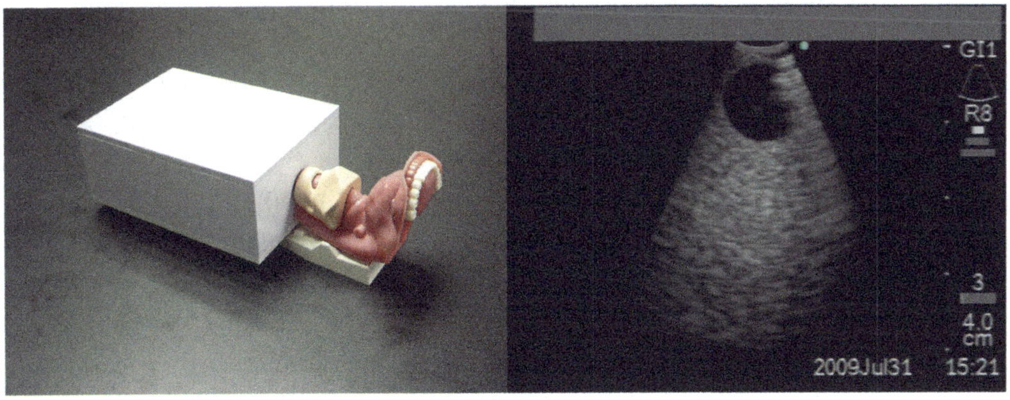

- Model constructed using a Laerdal upper airway and tracheal endoscopic ultrasound teaching phantom with bifurcation and non-echogenic structures (ATS laboratories Inc. Bridgeport CT)

Training Program

Informed Consent, Patient Safety, Procedural Pause (Time-Out)

Learning materials (Items 1-6 should be reviewed prior to workshop participation)

1. Informed consent/research and procedures: read the essay from The Picture of Health: Medical ethics and the movies (Oxford University Press). View film clip from *Extreme Measures.*

2. Informed consent/competence and capacity: read the essay from The Picture of Health: Medical ethics and the movies (Oxford University Press). View film clip from *A Beautiful Mind.*

3. Simulation session: read case descriptions, debriefing and concepts.

4. Read the manuscript *Psychological Aspects of Flexible Bronchoscopy* (by Colt, Goldman, Edell, and Knippa).

5. Read *Medical Informed Consent: general considerations for physicians* (by Patrick et al).

6. Read the text abstracted from *Institute for Clinical Systems Improvement* (ICSI) *Guidelines for safe site invasive procedures non-operating room,* downloaded from http://www.icsi.org/ January 2010.

7. Read the text abstracted from Center for Disease Control *CDC Universal Precautions* downloaded from cdc.gov January 2010.

8. Participation in group session simulation workshop (duration 90 minutes) during which materials are reviewed and case-based simulations pertaining to informed consent, patient safety, and procedural pause are performed.

9. Interactive session with critical review of a scene from the film *Death of Mr. Lazarescu.*

10. Interactive session (one-on-one assessment) with instructor for scoring and feedback purposes.

Informed Consent, Patient Safety, and Procedural Pause (Time-Out)*

Case Information

Part 1: Demographics

Case Title: Informed Consent, Patient Safety, Procedural Pause (Time Out)
Subject Name: (1) JJ (2) TL (3) DY
Scenario Name: Informed consent-patient safety-procedural pause
Simulation Developer(s): H. Colt
Date(s) of Development: September 2011

Appropriate for following learning groups

Post graduate education, Physicians in practice

Residents

Specialties: Pulmonary Anesthesiology Surgery Critical Care

Medical Students

Simulated patients 3 scenarios

Scenario # 1 (10 minutes, with 10 minutes debriefing): Obtain informed consent for EBUS-TBNA from a patient with suspected bronchogenic carcinoma and mediastinal adenopathy.

Scenario # 2 (10 minutes, with 10 minutes debriefing): Identify important elements of history and physical in a patient with coronary artery disease and hypertension being evaluated for EBUS-TBNA.

* Template for Simulation Patient. Design Modified from original template by *Jeffrey M. Taekman, M.D, Duke University Simulation and Patient Safety Center*

Scenario # 3 (10 minutes with 10 minutes debriefing): Review all of the elements of a Procedural Pause (Time Out) for a patient about to undergo EBUS-TBNA under general anesthesia.

Scenario description: The instructor will read the scenario to the team. A specially trained patient educator will be the subject of the simulation. A team member will be designated to lead the simulation, and together with other team members, the team will proceed to perform each of the scenarios with guidance and specific instruction from the instructor. It is assumed that approximately ten minutes will be devoted to each scenario, with 10 minutes for an instructor-led debriefing. The instructor may choose to perform a ten minutes debriefing after moving the team through each of the three scenarios.

Part 2: Curricular Information

Educational Rationale:

There has been little or no emphasis on methods for obtaining informed consent for interventional pulmonary procedures, including EBUS-TBNA. We believe that developing and applying guidelines for informed consent is necessary in view of the increasing number and complexity of interventional procedures to ensure that specific information about each procedure, as well as benefits, potential complications, and alternatives are shared with the patient. In addition, in an environment that respects cultural diversity, this information should be shared in respect with patient-defined goals, values and priorities, including participation of family members, when desired or warranted, in the information sharing and decision-making process.

Morbidity and mortality from medical errors is a growing concern for the public, and for healthcare professionals. Patient safety has become of outmost importance, especially in regards to interventional pulmonary diagnostic and therapeutic procedures, where, at least in the United States, where the legal system does not consider interventional pulmonologists to be practicing potentially dangerous or life-threatening procedures. Patient safety also includes knowledge and performance of the procedural pause, now mandatory in the Unites States in both the bronchoscopy suite and the operating room theater. We believe that it is possible to implement greater patient safety measures if bronchoscopists were regularly informed and instructed about these patient safety practices.

Learning Objectives:

- The learner should be able to characterize the informed consent process according to accepted criteria
- The learner should be able to characterize the informed consent process in the setting of an emergency airway procedure where interaction is only possible with a family member.
- The learner should be able to identify specific questions while obtaining the patient's history that help to ensure patient safety.
- The learner should be able to enumerate the elements of a procedural pause and lead the bronchoscopy healthcare team in a "time-out."

Guided Study Questions:

- What are the key elements of informed consent?
- In respect for cultural diversity, what elements should be taken into consideration?
- What key elements of the patient history are important for enhancing patient safety during an interventional diagnostic or therapeutic pulmonary procedure?
- What are the key elements of the procedural pause? Why is such a "time out" necessary?

References (in addition to those provided for this session)

- Braddock CH et al, How doctors and patients discuss routine clinical decisions. J. Gen Intern Med 1997;12:339-345
- Etchells E et al. Patient safety in surgery: error detection and prevention. World J Surg 2003;27:936-942.
- Colt HG. Functional evaluation before and after interventional bronchoscopy. In, Interventional Bronchoscopy, Prog Resp Research 2000; 30:55-65, Karger Eds.
- Joint Commission for the Accreditation of Healthcare Organizations. National Patient Safety Goals, 2006.
- ICSI Guidelines safe site invasive procedures non-operating room. Available fromhttp://www.guideline.gov/summary/summary.aspx?ss=15&doc_id=13702.

Didactics:

- Not applicable

Assessment Instruments:

- Informed consent checklist
- Procedural pause checklist
- Patient safety and procedure-related precautions checklist

Part 3: Preparation

Monitors Required:

Not applicable

Other equipment required:

Not applicable

Time Duration

For each scenario

Set-up	5 minutes
Preparation	2 minutes
Simulation	10 minutes
Debrief	10 minutes

Part 4: Supporting Files (case scenario handouts)

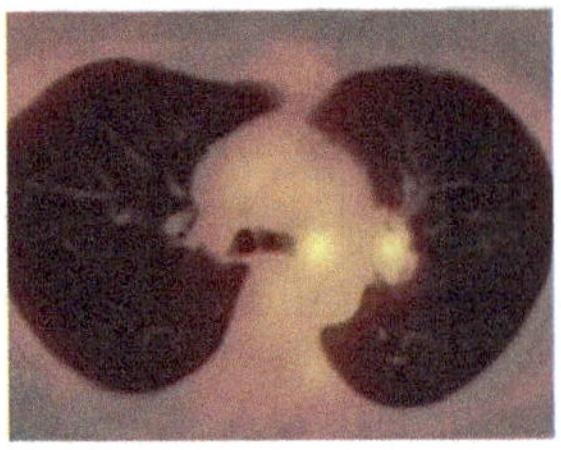

Scenario # 1 (Informed consent): A 74 year old male a history of weight loss has been diagnosed with a lung mass and mediastinal adenopathy on PET-CT. He is referred forEBUS-TBNA for diagnosis and possible staging.

You must obtain informed consent from the patient for EBUS-TBNA in order to determine the cause for these radiographic findings.

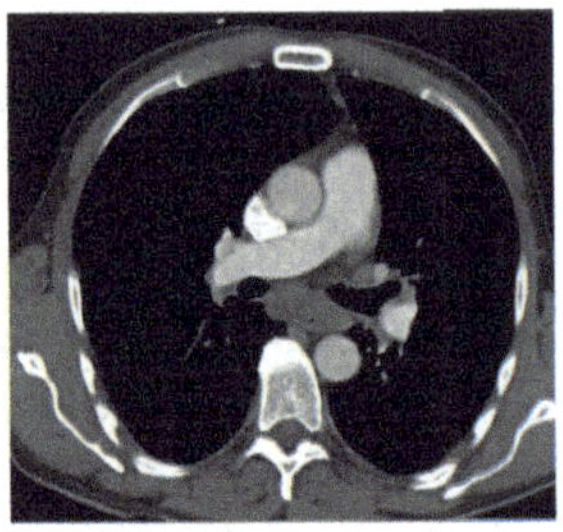

Scenario # 2 (Patient safety): A 50 year old Asian male with a history of chest pain, known coronary artery disease and systemic hypertension is referred for EBUS-TBNA of a large subcarinal lymph node. Previous flexible bronchoscopy and bronchoalveolar lavage were nondiagnostic.

In addition to obtaining informed consent, you must identify elements from the history that will help assure patient safety during and after the procedure.

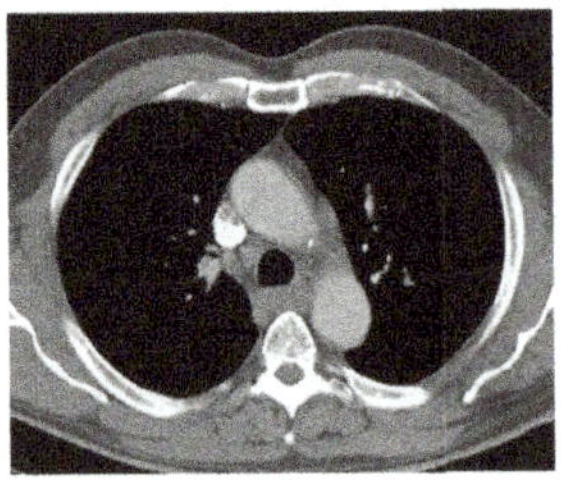

Scenario # 3 (Procedural pause): A 60 year old woman with known lung cancer and a history of tuberculosis currently on treatment is about to undergo EBUS-TBNA for staging purposes. She has a small right paratracheal lymph node. She has no known distant metastases. She is currently on the gurney in the operating room where she will be intubated for the procedure.

In addition to the procedural pause, you must identify procedure-related elements such as universal precautions, droplet precautions, and airborne pathogen precautions instituted, before, during and after the procedure.

Part 5: Debriefing

Scenario # 1: Informed Consent

Elements of informed decision making include: (1) discussion of the clinical issue, (2) description of the procedure, (3) discussion of the risks and potential benefits of the procedure, (4) discussion of the therapeutic alternatives, and potential consequences from choosing those alternatives, (5) discussion of the implications of declining treatment, (6) assessment of the patient's and/or family member's understanding, (7) discussion of the uncertainties associated with the decision, and (8) asking the patient and family to express a preference.

Scenario # 2: Patient Safety and Procedure-Related Precautions

Elements crucial to safe bronchoscopic intervention, moderate or deep sedation, and general anesthesia include (1) review of medical history such as COPD, pulmonary embolus, deep venous thrombosis, rheumatoid arthritis, ankylosing spondylitis , infectious lung disease, other illnesses potentially affecting the airway, cardiac disease, pacemaker, coronary artery disease, obstructive sleep apnea, CO2 retention, laryngospasm or bronchospasm, asthma; (2) review of surgical history such as neck surgery, lung surgery, spine surgery; (3) dentures or loose teeth that might interfere with appropriate response to procedure-related complications; (4) bleeding disorder; (5) allergies to medications including local anesthetics, antibiotics, or reactions to general anesthetic drugs; (6) medication usage including anticoagulation, antiplatelet agents or clopidogrel (Plavix); (7) living situation and family or friend support system; (8) proximity to medical center and physician services; (9) pregnancy; (10) inquiry regarding advanced directives and health care decision making. (12) Universal precautions should always be used to protect the patient and the health care team from spread of blood borne infections such as Hepatitis and HIV. (13) Droplet precautions are warranted in case of risk for infectious lung disease which are droplet-transmitted (14) Airborne pathogens precautions are warranted in selected cases, especially in case of suspicion for tuberculosis or influenza. (15) Resuscitation cart must always be readily available, regularly checked and restocked.

Scenario # 3: Procedural Pause (Time-Out)

The procedural pause is performed immediately prior to the start of a procedure and must include specific elements to assure patient safety and avoid wrong procedure-wrong site-wrong patient events. A visual memory (triggers) is helpful to assure that all elements are addressed. These include (1) verification of patient, (2) verification of procedure, (3) verification of site and side, (4) verification of consistency with signed informed consent, (5) verification of availability of medical records and equipment, (6) declaration of need for medication or fluids, (7) description of allergies, drug reactions, (8) declaration and communication regarding other safety concerns. Initiated by the team leader, a verbal acknowledgement is required by all members of the health care team. During the time-out, each person in the room should stop what they are doing and actively participate in the process. No individual is exempt, and active participation requires that each individual state clearly that they agree with the elements of the time-out. Any discrepancies and disagreements must be addressed before the procedure begins. If any distractions occur during the time-out, or if another individual enters the room or if a telephone rings, the time-out must be restarted.

****

Informed Consent Patient Safety and Time Out Slide Handout

INFORMED CONSENT

Bronchoscopy.org

Concept of Informed Consent

- Protects patient by providing information for informed decision-making
- Protects health care providers from liability provided procedure is executed according to prevailing standards and without negligence.
- Providers opportunity to consider and reconsider alternatives.
- Provides opportunity to discuss risks, benefits, and possible complications.

Bronchoscopy.org

Requirement for Informed Consent

- Must be informed and effective
- To be informed, a patient must be given information about the procedure relevant to their individual situation.
- To be effective, the person undergoing the procedure should be able to demonstrate in their own words, their understanding of the procedure or treatment.

Bronchoscopy.org

American Medical Association

- Informed consent is a "process" to discuss diagnosis and clinical issues
- As well as to discuss nature and purpose of proposed procedure., and its risks and benefits
- Discuss alternatives regardless of cost or insurance coverage, as well as potential risks and benefits of choosing an alternative
- Discuss risks and benefits of NOT receiving or undergoing the procedure.

Bronchoscopy.org

PATIENT SAFETY and PRECAUTIONS

Bronchoscopy.org

Universal Precautions

- Medical and surgical history, bleeding disorders, allergies, medications, pregnancy, living situation, proximity to physician services, advanced directivesand medical decision-making.
- Universal precautions should always be used to protect the patient and the health care team from spread of blood borne infections such as Hepatitis and HIV.
- Gloves, Hand-washing, Gowns, Surface disinfection, Sharp containers

Bronchoscopy.org

Droplet Precautions

- Droplet precautions are warranted in patients known or suspected to be infected with microorganisms transmitted by droplets (larger than 5 microns in size) that can be generated by coughing, sneezing, talking, or during the procedure.
  - Surgical masks, facial shield, or goggles
  - patient transport precautions
  - Droplet precaution sign on procedure room door
  - Cough/respiratory hygiene etiquette

Bronchoscopy.org

Airborne Pathogens Precautions

- Hand hygiene
- Cough/respiratory hygiene etiquette
- Cleaning and disinfection of contaminated surfaces
- Negative airflow with external exhaust
- N-95 respiratory or other National Institute for Occupational Safety and Health recommended device.
- Power air purifying respiratory (PAPR) might be considered in selected high risk cases.
- Airborne precautions sign

Bronchoscopy.org

PROCEDURAL PAUSE

Bronchoscopy.org

The concept of a "Procedural Pause", also known as a "Time Out"

- This safety protocol eliminates events involving the wrong patient, wrong site or wrong procedure.
- The protocol has been endorsed by more than fifty professional organizations, and is applicable to all high-risk procedures.
- The protocol is included in the USA Joint Commission for the Accreditation of Healthcare Organization National Patient Safety Goals project and was originally approved in 2004.
- The protocol also includes other components important in fostering a culture of patient safety, such as purposeful team communication and ensuring patient understanding.

Bronchoscopy.org

Requirements of an active "Time Out"

- Performed immediately prior to the start of the procedure.
- Ensures that the correct patient, site, positioning, and procedure to be performed are correctly identified.
- Ensures that pertinent imaging studies, medical records and equipment are available.
- Initiated by the provider and includes active verbal acknowledgement by all members of the health care team and any other persons present.
- All environmental distractions should be eliminated as much as possible.

Bronchoscopy.org

Time Out: visual memory guide

1. Verification of patient
   This is patient (read name badge), confirm with patient or family.
2. Verification of procedure "I am Dr….We are going to perform …Patient agrees…"
3. Verification of side and site
4. Nurse verifies consistency with signed informed consent.
5. Team members verify and declare availability of pertinent medical records, imaging studies and equipment.
6. Declare need for antibiotics, fluids or moderate sedation.
7. Describe allergies or drug reactions
8. Declare of safety issues based on medical history

Bronchoscopy.org

Informed Consent: A Summary of Policy and Process

Colt HG, Goldman AJ, Knippa J, and Edell E

The Process of Informed Consent

The concept of *Voluntary Informed Consent* has been studied by the American judicial system for a number of years[1]. It is the legal embodiment of the concept that each individual has the right to make decisions affecting his or her well-being[2]. The "Doctrine of Informed Consent" may have been originally derived from the 1947 Nuremberg Code which required that doctors obtain the voluntary informed consent of a subject prior to conducting medical experimentation. As a result of these Nuremberg trials, where it was discovered that Nazi doctors had performed grotesque medical experiments on prisoners and work camp detainees, Human Subjects Institutional Review Boards and ethics committees were also created, in part to protect the rights of both patients and research subjects, and to assure compliance with the subsequent 1964 World Medical Association's Declaration of Helsinki formulation of an international code of ethics to address concerns about the preservation of autonomy, beneficence, nonmaleficence, and justice for human research subjects[3].

The Informed Consent Doctrine requires that medical doctors provide a patient with all relevant information about a proposed procedure or treatment prior to obtaining the consent of the patient to carry out that procedure or treatment. Informed consent protects the patient by providing them with complete information on which to make an informed decision. Informed consent may also, at times, protect the health care provider from liability (with exceptions) provided that the procedure is properly executed according to the prevailing standards of care in the community and without negligence. In addition, the informed consent process gives health care providers and patients an opportunity to consider and re-consider the diagnostic and therapeutic strategies being proposed, as well as the possible risks and benefits of such procedures and to prepare, as needed, for procedure-related adverse events. From a patient's perspective, one might prepare for and lessen procedure-related anxiety by designating surrogate decision makers in case of procedure-related complications, assuring notification about advanced directives and code status, or by requesting the presence of family members at the time of the intervention.

From a legal standpoint, at least in the United States, consent for a medical procedure must be both *informed* and *effective.* To be *informed,* a person must be given information about the procedure relevant to their individual situation. To be *effective,* the person undergoing the procedure should be able to demonstrate, in his or her own words, their understanding of the procedure. Merely asking a person if they understand and receiving a "yes" or a head nod in response is generally considered insufficient. In some countries, informed consent needs to be documented by signatures from patients, witnesses, and health care providers on a specially-designed document approved for use by the institution's medical and risk management committees. The validity in court of such documents has been debated, however, and in some North American institutions, physicians may be counseled to additionally describe the informed consent process in their dictated preprocedure notes.

Informed consent, therefore, is more than simply requesting that a patient sign a written consent form. It is a *process of communication* between a patient and a physician that results in the patient's authorization or agreement to undergo a specific medical intervention. During this dialogue, the physician who is performing the procedure; not a delegated representative, should disclose and discuss: (i) The patient's diagnosis, if known, or the concerning clinical issues, (ii) the nature and purpose of the proposed treatment or procedure, (iii) the risks and benefits of the proposed treatment or procedure (iv) alternative treatments regardless of their costs or if covered by health insurance, (v) potential risks and benefits from choosing alternative treatments or procedures, and (vi) the risks and benefits of <u>not</u> receiving or undergoing a treatment or procedure.

The patient in turn, should be given the opportunity to ask any questions which they deem necessary to gain a better understanding of the procedure so that an informed decision can be made to proceed with or to refuse that particular course of medical intervention. Health care providers should assure that the patient has truly understood the elements of the procedure as well as the elements of the informed consent process. This can be done by asking the patient to repeat, in their own words, their understanding of the procedure. From an ethics perspective, physicians should be expected to disclose any conflicts of interest or compensation gained from the treatments or procedures performed [4].

In children (when a patient is under 18 years of age, unless married or otherwise considered to be an "emancipated minor") or if an adult patient is mentally or physically incompetent, incapacitated, or if no Health Care Directive exists, a parent or other guardian can usually give surrogate consent or "permission", assuming that the surrogate has decisional capacity and legal empowerment to give such consent for medical care and that the surrogate is acting with the patient's best interest in mind and according to what the patient would have wanted had the patient been able to participate in the decision-making process. In the United States, when there is no guardian, the provisions of Section 59 of the Guardianship and Administration Act of 1993 apply and consent must then be obtained from a spouse, including a legal de-facto spouse, a parent, a sibling over 18 years of age, a son or daughter over 18 years of age, or a person (not being the guardian) who acts *in loco parentis.*

In emergency situations, a physician can proceed without obtaining consent when treatment is needed urgently to save a person's life or to prevent serious damage to a person's health and (i) the treating health care provider does not have any knowledge of a prior refusal by the person to the treatment, (ii) the patient has not appointed a Medical Agent, (iii) the patient has not appointed an Enduring Guardian, and (iv) there is no Guardianship Order with a guardian appointed by a Guardianship Board. Surprisingly, there is often very little difference between consent forms used for elective versus emergency procedures. In some cases, the content of these forms does not even meet the accepted standards of information delivery [5]. In addition, during emergencies, attention is not often given to an individual's level of understanding of their illness or, in some cases, to that individual's ability to even read or truly comprehend the informed consent form that they are expected to sign.

Informed Consent, Capacity, Competence, and the Law

The informed consent process in the United States and in most other countries is designed to ensure not only the satisfaction of legal, ethical, and accreditation requirements, but also the *quality* and *safety* of patient treatments and procedures. A patient's right to informed consent or to refuse a medical treatment or procedure can thus be enforced in a number of ways, including through state common law, federal and state statutes and regulations, medical ethics, and Joint Commission hospital guidelines.

Studies outside of the realm of bronchoscopy have shown that even after consent is obtained, 18% to 45% of patients cannot state the major risks associated with their procedures [6]. It is unclear whether this is the result of poor communication, lack of information, poor recall as a consequence of procedure-related stress and anxiety, or absence of memory reinforcement. At least one study has shown that patients who are simply asked to recount what they have learned during the informed consent discussion have greater recall and comprehension of that interaction than those who are not asked to recount the interaction [7]. A written and signed consent form, while not replacing the discussion between a patient and their provider, supports legal evidence such as testimony and notes in the medical record, of the validity of the patient's informed and agreed upon understandings and statements concerning the procedure.

Underlying the concept of informed consent is the assumption that a patient is cognitively competent. From the sociological standpoint, *competence* is defined as having sufficient ability to make choices such that personal autonomy remains intact. Legally, *competence* is a state in which an individual's decision-making ability is adequate to meet the demands of a clearly specified decision-making task. A person may therefore be competent in some endeavors but not in others. Based on a review of judicial opinions and case law in the United States, legal standards of competence to consent to procedures include the ability to understand the information that is provided, the ability to appreciate one's own situation in light of the information provided, the ability to reason with the information provided, and the ability to express a choice. Curiously, only the abilities to understand information and to express a choice are universally held as legal standards upon which to base a determination of competence [8].

Technically, medical professionals lack the legal authority to determine competence, and instead are able to determine whether a patient has decision-making *capacity*. A patient may, for example, be capable of making the decision to refuse to undergo a procedure, yet be found legally incompetent to handle their personal finances. Often, a physician's assessment of decision-making capacity guides legal determinations of competence, and it is frequently the physician's finding of incapacity that causes alternative forms of consent to be sought, and a patient's legal rights to be temporarily suspended without involvement of the courts.

It seems reasonable to question whether voluntary choice and decisional competence and capacity are truly preserved in a medical emergency. There are considerable barriers, conscious and unconscious, as well as intellectual and emotional, to assimilating information during an acute illness, trauma, or life-threatening event. It is generally accepted that patients who have received sedatives or narcotics as part of a treatment plan for respiratory insufficiency, intubation, pain, or high-grade anxiety should not be asked for permission to perform invasive procedures.

Sometimes, even the stress of illness may suffice to alter the decision-making capacities of otherwise reasonable individuals. Studies of patients with acute myocardial infarctions, for example, suggest that psychological or physical stress alone may compromise understanding [9-13]. Assessments of decisional abilities before a determination of capacity can be reached are also difficult in patients with suspected neurologic or cognitive impairment accompanied by communicative dysfunction, especially when there is limited time in which to institute a treatment plan; for example, when emergency intubation is required for survival (note that as of this writing, there is no validated instrument for measuring cognitive and procedure-related decision-making capacity in patients with acute stroke).

References

1. Berg JW, Appelbaum PJ. *Informed consent: legal theory and clinical practice.* 2nd ed. New York, Oxford University Press Inc. 2001.
2. Merz JF. An Empirical Analysis of the Medical Informed Consent Doctrine; Search for a "Standard of Disclosure *httpllwww.peircelaw.edulvo2lwinterlmerz.htm;* pp 1-27.
3. Declaration of Helsinki. Downloaded from http://www.wma.net/e/policy/b3.htm. Accessed, November 20, 2008.
4. Colt HG and Mulnard RA. Writing an application for a human subjects institutional review board. *Chest.* 2006;130:1605-1607.
5. Bottrell MM, Fischback AH, Emanuel LL; Hospital Informed Consent Forms: Facilitating Quality patient-physician Interaction. *Arch Surg.* 2000;135(1):23-26.
6. Beckman HB, Merkakis KM, Suchman AL, Frankel RM; The Doctor-Patient Relationship and Malpractice Lessons from Plaintiff Depositions. *Arch Intern Med.* 1994;154:1365-1370.
7. Claims RX: Clinical and Risk Management Perspectives; Informed Consent Update; The NORCAL Mutual Insurance Company Newsletter; March, 2007.
8. White-Bateman SR, Schumacher C, Sacco RL, Appelbaum PS; Consent for Intravenous Thrombolysis in Acute Stoke. *Arch Neurol.* 2007;64:785-792.
9. Agard A, Hermeren G, Herlitz J. Patient's Experiences of Intervention Trials on the Treatment of Myocardial Infarction: Is it Time to Adjust the Informed Consent Procedure to the Patient's Capacity? *Heart.* 2001;86:632-637.
10. Williams BF, French JK, White HD; Is Our Method of Obtaining Consent Appropriate for Randomised Controlled Trials in Acute Myocardial Infarction? *NZ Med J.* 1997;110:298-299.
11. Schmidt TA, Salo SD, Hughes JA, et al; SAEM Ethics Committee. Confronting the Ethical Challenges to Informed Consent in Emergency Medicine Research. *Acad Emerg Med.* 2004;11:1082-1089.
12. Akkad A, Jackson C, Dixon-Wood M, Taub N Habiba M; Informed Consent for Elective and Emergency Surgery; Questionnaire Study. *BJOG.* 2004;111:1133-1138.
13. Kondziolka DS, Pirris SM, Lunsford LD; Improving the Informed Consent Process for Surgery. *Neurosurgery.* 2006;58 (1):1184-1189.

****

Excerpt from *Extreme Measures* & Informed Consent

The Picture of Health: Medical Ethics and Movies (Oxford University Press 2011)

Henri Colt M.D. FCCP (with permission)

Extreme Measures (1996). Hugh Grant, Gene Hackman, Sarah Jessica Parker. Directed by Michael Apted. Duration 120 minutes.

DVD Chapter 34 Scene 01:43:25 to 01:45:00

Extreme Measures tells the story of Dr. Guy Luthan (Hugh Grant), an Emergency Room physician entering a Neurology Fellowship in a New York Hospital. Luthan faces issues of conscience and professionalism after one of his patients, a homeless man with an identification wristband from a hospital Luthan has never heard of, dies and the body disappears. As he begins inquiries into the incident, he meets world-renowned Dr. Lawrence Myrick (Gene Hackman), a neurosurgeon who performs experimental spinal surgeries on the homeless in an attempt to find a cure to paralyzing spinal disorders.

In this scene, it appears that surgery has been performed without consent in physically fit, homeless individuals. The major protagonist of these actions. Dr. Myrick, declares that he is 68 years old, and does not have time to do experiments first in rats, then in chimpanzees. He further justifies human experimentation in nonconsenting, uninformed individuals by saying that great advances in medical science can only occur when physicians do what they think is right, even if it involves breaking rules. "People die every day," he says, "And for what? For nothing. What do we do?What do you do? You take care of the ones you think you can save. Good doctors do the correct thing, but great doctors have the guts to do the right thing".

I often use the plot lines of *Extreme Measures* as springboards for discussions about informed consent, and more recently, about the appropriateness of incorporating a "time out" prior to any surgical intervention in order to help avoid performing inappropriate surgeries or operating on the wrong patient. With respect first to the surgery without consent issue, one needs to understand the legal notions of assault and battery. These were highlighted in the landmark case of *Schloendorff v Society of New York* regarding a surgeon who had performed a hysterectomy without consent. The law, which is based on the principle of self-determination[1], states that a person has the right to remain free from aggression against one's person.

From a legal perspective, *Assault* consists of a bodily threat and ability to do harm without a person's consent. Certainly, a surgeon has the ability to do harm either by operating inappropriately on a consenting patient, by performing procedures on a nonconsenting patient, and by performing the wrong procedure. Health care providers might also threaten to do harm by insisting on the performance of a procedure against a patient's wishes. *Battery*, on the other-hand, consists of any intentional bodily contact that violates the personal physical security of another without that person's permission. The batter victim does not need to be aware that physical violation has occurred. Such a scenario would apply to a patient who has been sedated or rendered unconscious by anesthesia. Nor do battery charges require that actual damage be demonstrated.

From a historical perspective, the doctrine of informed consent seems to have derived from the 1947 Nuremberg Code. This required doctors to obtain voluntary informed consent prior to conducting medical experimentation, and declared that all relevant information about a proposed procedure or treatment be provided prior to obtaining such consent. As a result of the Nuremberg trials, where it was discovered that Nazi doctors had performed grotesque medical experiments on prisoners and work camp detainees, Human Subjects Institutional Review Boards (IRBs) were created, in part to protect the rights of both patients and research subjects. With the World Medical Association's Declaration of Helsinki in 1964, an international code of ethics was also formulated to address concerns about the preservation of autonomy, beneficence, nonmaleficence, and justice for all human research subjects[2].

Institutional Review Boards (IRBs) oversee research protocols, monitor drug and treatment trials, and help investigators maintain appropriate records in case of inquiry[3]. In the United States, the Code of Federal Regulations Protection of Human Subjects (45CFR Part 46), is actually a direct result of various abuses of patient rights, such as those that occurred during the 30-year government-sponsored Tuskegee syphilis study, during which 300 black men were untreated despite the recognized effectiveness of antibiotic treatment. Today, one of the roles of an IRB is to assure that informed consent documents are written in such a way that all potential research subjects are able to understand the risks and benefits of any proposed research[4].

The American Medical Association has opinioned, however, that informed consent entails more than just informing patents about the risks and benefits of a proposed intervention or research project. It is a process of communication between a patient and a physician that results in the patient's authorization and agreement to undergo a specific medical intervention, ensuring that the patient has truly understood the elements of the procedure, as well as the consequences of undergoing or refusing to undergo the intervention[5]. It follows that physicians must disclose any and all conflicts of interest or compensation gained from any treatments or research being proposed. Similar recommendations have been issued by the British Medical Association, with emphasis on a patient-centered model of care whereby physicians are encouraged to take into consideration a patient's goals, values, and objectives and to provide information accordingly[6,7].

While the Nuremberg Code insisted on consent from research subjects, subsequent arguments have been made that in the case of therapeutic procedures on incompetent patients, and in research patients for whom there are no effective therapies, a strict requirement for informed consent may be viewed as contrary to the subject's best interests. Obviously, this argument cannot and should not be made in relation to this film, because the subjects of the experimental research in *Extreme Measures* are neither incompetent, nor are they the persons with disease. The film thus prompts one to ask whether the research might have been justified if it were being performed on those individuals with neurological injuries, rather than on the unwilling, disenfranchised, healthy, homeless subjects. Considering the ethical principles of autonomy, nonmaleficence, and a health care provider's duty to obtain informed consent, the answer to this question is a resounding no.

Regardless of place or type of medical practice, respect for individual autonomy mandates the informed consent process. Whether health care interventions occur from within a patient-focused or family-focused care model, informed consent is representative of shared decision making. Informed consent, as well as recently mandated surgical "time out" rules, helps ensure the satisfaction of legal and ethical obligations, and enhance the quality and safety of patient treatments and procedures[8].

In addition, the health care provider's duties to do no harm reasonably trump any arguments that might be presented to justify assault and battery in the clinical setting. In cases where there is a need for emergency intervention in incompetent patients, or in cases where patients are without decision making capacity and surrogate consent cannot be obtained, however, procedures might be performed on condition that patients could potentially benefit and that patient acceptance would be probable.

In *Extreme Measures*, however, justifications for performing surgery on individuals without their consent include the necessity to proceed with human experimentation because the results would benefit paralyzed patients. Another way to ponder some of the ethical dilemmas facing the health care providers in the film, as well as their administrative staff, therefore, is to reflect whether a common good (beneficence for society, or, in this case, specifically to the spinal disorders patient community), might in fact, warrant the physical, emotional, and psychological harm done to the unwilling study subject. This is counter, of course, to the principles of respect for autonomy and need to provide medical care while safeguarding a patient's best interests.

On the other hand, from a simple philosophical utilitarian perspective, one might argue that a greater good is accomplished for society as a whole, and that the disenfranchised study subjects provide no benefit to society other than their availability as objects of experimentation. If such an argument is deemed unacceptable, it is curious that similar perspectives are proposed to help justify the use and abuse of animals in research and procedural-based education, or the ready accessibility to patients, rather than to more costly inanimate and computer-based simulation in order to help health care providers improve their diagnostic and therapeutic procedural technical skills. In *Extreme Measures*, Myrick tells Luthan that the homeless persons undergoing experimental surgical procedures without consent, are, in fact, heroes because losing one to save millions is worthy of their sacrifice.

References

1. James L. Bernat, Lynn M. Peterson," Patient-centered informed consent in surgical practice," *Arch Surg* 141 (2006):86-92.
2. Declaration of Helsinki. Downloaded from http://www.wma.net/e/policy/b3.htm. Accessed, (November 20, 2008).
3. Robert A. Greenwald, Mary Kay Ryan, James E Mulvihill, *Human subjects research: A handbook for institutional review boards* (New York: Plenum Press, 1982).
4. Henri G. Colt, Ruth A Mulnard," Writing for a Human Subjects Institutional Review Board," *Chest* 130 (2006):1605-1607.
5. Council on Ethical and Judicial Affairs, *American Medical Association Code of Ethics,* 1st ed. (Chicago: American Medical Association, 2008)

6. Len Doyal, Jeffrey S. Tobias, eds. "Informed consent in medical research," *BMJ* 316 (March 28, 1998): 1000-5
7. John Bridson, Clare Hammond, Austin Leach, Michael R. Chester," Making consent patient centered," *BMJ* 327 (November 15, 2003):1159-1161.
8. Jessica W. Berg, Paul S. Appelbaum, *Informed consent: legal theory and clinical practice*, 2nd ed. (New York: Oxford University Press Inc, 2001).

****

Excerpt from *A Beautiful Mind* & Informed Consent

The Picture of Health: Medical Ethics and Movies (Oxford University Press 2011)

Jay A. Jacobson, M.D., MACP (with permission)

A Beautiful Mind (2001). Russell Crowe, Jennifer Connelly, Christopher Plummer
Directed by Ron Howard. Duration: 136 minutes

DVD chapter 16, Scene 01.39.05 to 01.42.30

A Beautiful Mind, inspired by a true story, explores the life, real and imagined, of John Nash Jr. (Russell Crowe) who is a brilliant, ultimately Nobel Prize winning mathematician, but who develops schizophrenia. His mind, still beautiful, but now untrustworthy, is capable of solving even previously insoluble theoretical problems, but is not always capable of distinguishing reality from paranoid delusions and visual and auditory hallucinations. His medical treatment consisted of insulin shock treatments and an orally administered drug, both accompanied by significant adverse effects. The drug, however, was somewhat effective in controlling the symptoms of schizophrenia. Based on a delusional preoccupation with a conspiracy and his negative experience with treatment, Nash subsequently rejects treatment which leads to nearly catastrophic consequences. Ultimately, forced or, at least, coerced treatment and his heroic will and capacity to compartmentalize and separate reality from fantasy enable Professor Nash to pursue his passion for mathematics, manage his life and relationships, and do the complex work that eventually earns him international acclaim.

On a windy morning when John is responsible for bathing their baby, his wife, Alicia (Jennifer Connelly) steps outside to bring in clothes hanging on the line. The sound of a radio and a banging door draw her to the shed where she is shocked by evidence of John's unabated schizophrenic delusions. Realizing that he is not taking his drug and fearful for the baby's safety, she rushes back inside the house, finds and rescues the frightened, crying baby from a tub rapidly filling with water. Actively hallucinating, John imagines that his wife's call to his doctor constitutes a threat and knocks her down with their baby.

In the critical scene, Dr. Rosen has come to the Nash home. John admits that he stopped his medicine because of its side effects and he acknowledges persistent visual hallucinations. Dr. Rosen warns him that, if untreated, schizophrenia will only worsen and he recommends readmission to the hospital for more insulin shock and drug therapy. John is reluctant to begin another traumatic hospitalization that he fears will never end. Dr. Rosen has commitment papers which Alicia can sign that mandate admission and treatment. John hopes that she won't sign and wishes for more time to work this problem out. He affirms the doctor's judgment that "I'm not safe anymore". When Alicia asks him if he would hurt her, he says, "I don't know".

This scene illustrates the problem posed by the multi-tiered concept of informed consent, especially in the context of mental illness where decision making capacity and competence are especially hard to isolate and evaluate. The policy and practice of voluntary informed consent arose in response to forced, experimental and even lethal treatment of prisoners in Nazi concentration camps. We follow this practice in clinical settings as well. We grant patients with the mental capacity to make decisions a near absolute right to do so. We expect physicians to provide ample information and permit unforced consent or refusal. They should explain the indications for a treatment, its risks and benefits and the comparative results of treatment, alternative treatment, and no treatment.

One prerequisite for voluntary informed consent is an environment free of a compelling force that will drive the decision in one direction and negate the patient's ability and freedom to choose. Another is the mental capacity to make a reasoned choice. One way to assess this capacity is to establish if the patient has a set of values and goals, if the patient can communicate and understand information and can reason and deliberate about the choice.

In this scene, we have a physician who makes an assessment and recommends the medically indicated treatment. He predicts what will happen without treatment. He doesn't address side effects, but also does not dispute the observations that John makes about the negative effects of drug treatment. John has prior personal experience with the risks and benefits of treatment. Thus, to some extent the "informed" criteria for voluntary informed consent are met. What remains to be considered is whether John Nash, with his undeniable mental capacity for mathematical problem solving, has the mental capacity to make a reasonable and uncoerced personal treatment decision. If he lacks this capacity, others with his best interest in mind, can and should make the choice for him. If he has the capacity and refuses the therapy that others think best for him are there valid and ethical reasons to override that choice?

John, even in his unmedicated, self-acknowledged delusional state does seem to have sustained values and goals. His goal is to pursue his professional work, to solve problems. He values knowledge and his emotional attachment to his wife and child. He is able to communicate and understand information from the doctor, although he reaches a different conclusion about treatment. Unfortunately, we've seen that he can't reliably discriminate between information coming from a real or an imagined source. He does seem to be able to reason about and give reasons for his choices. His belief about the result of another hospi- talization demonstrates his ability to connect an intervention with an outcome even if the outcome he foresees may not be the positive one that the doctor and Alicia are hoping for. It is a possible and plausible outcome.

A person's ability to make decisions is both ethically and legally important. In law, it permits individuals to make choices, even those judged unwise by others, and it makes individuals responsible for intentional actions that break laws or harm others. In medical ethics, it is the basis for providing relevant information to patients prior to treatment or procedures and for respecting their decision to proceed or refuse. Legal cases about cognitive ability often arise in the context of financial matters, reproductive choices or crimes. Medical ethics discussions of this ability usually pertain to decisions that affect the individual's health. The law presumes that individuals acquire sufficient decision-making ability when they become adults. The age of adulthood, rather than some demonstrated ability, becomes the standard and is set by statute. The law regards adults, absent evidence to the contrary, to be able and entitled to make their own decisions. The legal term for this is competent. Adults retain the right to make a full range of decisions for themselves unless a judge-rules, based on evidence, that they are incompetent. Medical ethics is attentive to context and to individual differences in ability. In emergencies, for example, when medical decisions must be made quickly, if patients are temporarily mentally impaired or even unconscious, physicians generally proceed with treatment despite their patient's impaired or absent decision-making capacity. This is justified by the concept of implied consent.

When an adult patient's condition is not emergent and life threatening the law and medical ethics agree that consent for treatment is imperative. For patients who are obviously and permanently impaired who don't refuse treatment, physicians turn to family members to make the decision they believe the patient would have made or, if that's unknown, the decision that would be best for the patient. When patients, who have been functioning independently and making their own decisions, refuse treatment for a dangerous and serious condition, doctors and concerned family members understandably question the patient's ability and right to make what seems to them to be an irrational and self destructive decision. Before they can force an expressly unwanted medical intervention, physicians should attempt to understand the patient's reasons and capacity to make such decisions.

This medical assessment could be as simple as asking the patient five questions: What is the medical problem? What treatment has been recommended? What will happen to you with and without the treatment? Finally, what is the reason for the decision? Patients with decision making capacity demonstrate a correct understanding of the nature of the medical problem, its treatment and prognosis, and have a reason for the decision. When such patients offer a reason that seems irrational and unconnected with a personal, religious, or cultural set of beliefs and values, a more expert evaluation by a mental health professional is appropriate. The expert may conclude that the patient, even though mentally or emotionally ill, has the capacity to make medical decisions. If this expert decides the patient lacks decision making capacity, the patient or someone on his behalf may still assert his legal competence and right to refuse treatment. If the patient appears to be a threat to himself or others, clinicians can temporarily take steps such as hospitalization to address that danger. However, to continue this beyond two or three days or begin treatment will require that a legal determination of competence be made.

Based on her questions to the patient, information from the family, and the opinion of experts, a judge decides whether a patient is competent. If so, the patient retains his right to refuse treatment. If not, the judge will appoint someone to be the guardian and decision maker for the patient. This could be a family member or someone specifically chosen for this task.

The film, *A Beautiful Mind*, doesn't include a legal determination of competence and it is ambiguous about whether John Nash is ultimately persuaded or voluntarily chooses medical treatment. Fortunately for him and for the viewers he somehow becomes able to manage the symptoms of his mental illness and resume a meaningful professional and family role. A patient's mental illness and impaired decision making often cause physicians and family members to feel frustration as they try to do what they believe is best for patients, but encounter what they view as legal obstacles. The law, however, is there to safeguard competent patients' rights and protect their liberty to make even seemingly unwise decisions. The law does balance the rights of individuals to decide against the consequences of their decision for others. Interestingly, even competent patients may have their liberty curtailed if they refuse treatment for a readily communicated serious disease such as tuberculosis. Thus, imminent danger to others and self is a reason for hospitalization or institutionalization that doctors, families, and judges can all agree on.

When diseases are dire and their treatments are safe, simple, well tolerated, inexpensive, highly effective and life-saving, doctors zealously advocate for them and most patients accept their recommendation. When we develop fully effective, better tolerated treatments for mental illnesses such as schizophrenia, patients may be more willing to accept them and thus help us avoid the ethically, legally, and emotionally fraught decision to force treatment.

References

1. Applebaum PS. Assessment of patients' competence to consent to treatment. *N Engl J Med 2007*; 357:1834-1840.
2. Brock DW, Wartman SA. When competent patients make irrational choices. *N Engl J Med* 1990;323:1353-1355.
3. Grisso T, Appelbaum PS. *Assessing Competence to Consent to Treatment: A Guide for Physicians and Other Health Professionals*. NY, NY. Oxford University Press, 1998.
4. Kim SYH. When does decisional impairment become decisional incompetence? Ethical and methodological issues in capacity research in schizophrenia. *Schizophr Bull* 2006;32:92-97.
5. President's Commission for the Study of Ethical Problems in Medicine and Biomedical and Behavioral Research. *Making health care decisions*: a report on the ethical and legal implications of informed consent in the patient practitioner relationship. Vol 1. Washington, DC: Government Printing Office, 1982.

Time Out also known as Procedural Pause*

Abstracted from Institute for Clinical Systems Improvement Guidelines: safe site invasive procedures non-operating room. Downloaded ICSI.org, February 1, 2010 from http://www.guideline.gov/summary/summary.aspx?ss=15&doc_id=13702

Active oral Time Out process

The Time Out is to be performed immediately prior to the start of the procedure and is the final safety stop before the procedure is begun. The purpose of the Time Out is to ensure that the correct patient, site, side, positioning and procedure to be performed are all correctly verified. In addition, it is an opportunity to validate that any related images, equipment or implants are available.

The Time Out is to be initiated by the provider and includes active verbal acknowledgment by all members of the team. The scalpel, needle or other cutting/incising device is not to be handed to the provider until the Time Out has been completed. While it is desirable to actively include the patient in the Time Out, it is not always possible, particularly if the patient is under the influence of sedating medications or is otherwise unable to participate.

It is recommended that a visual memory aid be used to trigger the initiation of the Time Out. For example, a "Time Out" sign or towel can be used to cover the scalpel, needle or cutting/incising device as a reminder to conduct the Time Out. When one of these aids is used, it is important to hand it off the sterile field at the conclusion of the Time Out so there is no potential for it to become retained in the patient.

Every Time Out must include the following standard elements:

- Patient identity, using a minimum of two identifiers
- Procedure(s) to be performed (including internal and/or external laterality, multiples and/or level)
- Patient positioning if not already verified
- Procedure side, site and/or level including visualization of the provider's initials if applicable
- As appropriate, imaging, equipment, implants or special requirements (e.g., pre-procedure antibiotic administration)

The provider may delegate the Time Out elements to the nurse or other member of the team, but the initiation of the Time Out should be the responsibility of the provider. The nurse or other team member may refer to the patient consent for the Time Out elements. However, prior to its use, the consent must have been validated against other documents, such as history and physical, radiology or pathology reports, progress notes, etc.

During the Time Out, each person in the procedure room must stop what he or she is doing and actively participate in the process. Involved staff may include the provider, resident, student, anesthesia, scrub, nurse and/or vendors whenever present. No individual is exempt from the process. Active participation requires each individual to state clearly and loudly that they agree with the elements of the Time Out. The scalpel, needle or other cutting/incising device is not to be handed to the provider until the Time Out has been completed. If a member of the team refuses to actively participate in the Time Out, the scalpel, needle or cutting/incising device is not handed to the provider until that individual is replaced and the Time Out completed.

Environmental distractions are to be eliminated as much as possible during the Time Out. For example, music is turned off, pagers are set on vibrate, talking other than participation in Time Out ceases and no staff are permitted to enter or exit the room. If during the Time Out an interruption or distraction occurs (pager goes off or an individual enters the room), the Time Out must be restarted.

Additional Time Outs are to be performed when there are two or more different procedures performed on the same patient during the same procedure period, whether or not the procedures involve a new procedure team. The process and elements of the Time Out as described above must occur prior to the start of the next procedure.

If the patient needs to be repositioned during the procedure and this repositioning affects the patient's presentation (i.e., the patient is turned prone), an abbreviated Time Out including the site, side, level and/or visualization of the provider's initials will be conducted. The Time Out process will be the same as described above (e.g., elimination of distractions, active participation).

****

Universal Precautions

Excerpt from the Fact Sheet Center for Disease Control: Provided for informational and educational use only Downloaded February 1, 2010, from http://www.cdc.gov/ncidod/dhqp/bp_universal_precautions.html#

"Universal precautions," as defined by CDC, are a set of precautions designed to prevent transmission of human immunodeficiency virus (HIV), hepatitis B virus (HBV), and other bloodborne pathogens when providing first aid or health care. Under universal precautions, blood and certain body fluids of all patients are considered potentially infectious for HIV, HBV and other bloodborne pathogens.

Universal precautions took the place of and eliminated the need for the isolation category "Blood and Body Fluid Precautions" in the 1983 CDC Guidelines for Isolation Precautions in Hospitals. However, implementing universal precautions does not eliminate the need for other isolation precautions, such as droplet precautions for influenza, airborne isolation for pulmonary tuberculosis, or contact isolation for methicillin-resistant *Staphylococcus aureus.*

Universal precautions apply to blood, other body fluids containing visible blood, semen, and vaginal secretions. Universal precautions also apply to tissues and to the following fluids: cerebrospinal, synovial, pleural, peritoneal, pericardial, and amniotic fluids. Universal precautions do not apply to feces, nasal secretions, sputum, sweat, tears, urine, and vomitus unless they contain visible blood. Universal precautions do not apply to saliva except when visibly contaminated with blood or in the dental setting where blood contamination of saliva is predictable.

Universal precautions involve the use of protective barriers such as gloves, gowns, aprons, masks, or protective eyewear, which can reduce the risk of exposure of the health care worker's skin or mucous membranes to potentially infective materials. In addition, under universal precautions, it is recommended that all health care workers take precautions to prevent injuries caused by needles, scalpels, and other sharp instruments or devices.

Pregnant health care workers are not known to be at greater risk of contracting HIV infection than are health care workers who are not pregnant; however, if a health care worker develops HIV infection during pregnancy, the infant is at risk of infection resulting from perinatal transmission. Because of this risk, pregnant health care workers should be especially familiar with, and strictly adhere to, precautions to minimize the risk of HIV transmission.

GLOVING, GOWNING, MASKING, AND OTHER PROTECTIVE BARRIERS

All health care workers should routinely use appropriate barrier precautions to prevent skin and mucous membrane exposure during contact with any patient's blood or body fluids that require universal precautions.

Recommendations for the use of gloves are presented in detail in the Morbidity and Mortality Weekly Report dated June 24, 1988, which is available by calling the National AIDS Information Hotline at 1-800-342-2437 or the National AIDS Information Clearinghouse at 1-800-458-5231.

Gloves should be worn:

- for touching blood and body fluids requiring universal precautions, mucous membranes, or non-intact skin of all patients, and
- for handling items or surfaces soiled with blood or body fluids to which universal precautions apply.

Gloves should be changed after contact with each patient. Hands and other skin surfaces should be washed immediately or as soon as patient safety permits if contaminated with blood or body fluids requiring universal precautions. Hands should be washed immediately after gloves are removed. Gloves should reduce the incidence of blood contamination of hands during phlebotomy, but they cannot prevent penetrating injuries caused by needles or other sharp instruments. Institutions that judge routine gloving for all phlebotomies is not necessary should periodically reevaluate their policy. Gloves should always be available to health care workers who wish to use them for phlebotomy. In addition, the following general guidelines apply:

1. Use gloves for performing phlebotomy when the health care worker has cuts, scratches, or other breaks in his/her skin.
2. Use gloves in situations where the health care worker judges that hand contamination with blood may occur, e.g., when performing phlebotomy on an uncooperative patient.
3. Use gloves for performing finger and/or heel sticks on infants and children.
4. Use gloves when persons are receiving training in phlebotomy.

Masks and protective eyewear or face shields should be worn by health care workers to prevent exposure of mucous membranes of the mouth, nose, and eyes during procedures that are likely to generate droplets of blood or body fluids requiring universal precautions. Gowns or aprons should be worn during procedures that are likely to generate splashes of blood or body fluids requiring universal precautions.

All health care workers should take precautions to prevent injuries caused by needles, scalpels, and other sharp instruments or devices during procedures; when cleaning used instruments; during disposal of used needles; and when handling sharp instruments after procedures. To prevent needlestick injuries, needles should not be recapped by hand, purposely bent or broken by hand, removed from disposable syringes, or otherwise manipulated by hand. After they are used, disposable syringes and needles, scalpel blades, and other sharp items should be placed in puncture-resistant containers for disposal. The puncture-resistant containers should be located as close as practical to the use area. All reusable needles should be placed in a puncture-resistant container for transport to the reprocessing area.

General infection control practices should further minimize the already minute risk for salivary transmission of HIV. These infection control practices include the use of gloves for digital examination of mucous membranes and endotracheal suctioning, handwashing after exposure to saliva, and minimizing the need for emergency mouth-to-mouth resuscitation by making mouthpieces and other ventilation devices available for use in areas where the need for resuscitation is predictable.

****

EBUS Airway Access and Image Acquisition

Case Information

Part 1: Demographics

Case Title: Airway access and image acquisition
Subject Name: (1) Eddie Ebus
Scenario Name: Airway access and image acquisition
Simulation Developer(s): H. Colt
Date(s) of Development: September 2022

Appropriate for following learning groups

Post graduate education, Physicians in practice
Specialties: Pulmonary, Anesthesiology, Surgery, Critical Care
Thoracic surgeons performing EBUS

Simulated patient 1 scenario

Scenario # 1 (10 minutes, with 10 minutes debriefing): Access the airway using the 30-degree field of view EBUS bronchoscope through an oral airway, a Laryngeal Mask Airway and an endotracheal tube. Then demonstrate controls on the Ultrasound image processor including on/off switch, Gain, Depth, Color Doppler, Frequency, and measurement calipers.

Scenario description: The instructor will read the scenario to the team. It may be necessary for the instructor to demonstrate airway access techniques and image processor controls to the team. The learner will then proceed to access the airway using three techniques. After the third technique, and with the EBUS bronchoscope inside the EBUS model, the learner will demonstrate use of the image processor controls for altering the quality of the ultrasound image. It may be necessary to use more than one model for this exercise (an intubation head for airway access for example, and the EBUS box trainer with bifurcated airway and lymph node stations 2,4 and 7 for the image acquisition portion of the simulation). It is assumed that approximately ten minutes will be devoted to the scenario, with 10 minutes for an instructor-led debriefing. The instructor may further choose to perform an additional ten minutes debriefing that could include viewing the EBUS Physics instructional video.

* Template for Simulation Patient. Design Modified from original template by *Jeffrey M. Taekman, M.D, Duke University Simulation and Patient Safety Center*

Part 2: Curricular Information

Educational Rationale:

While airway access is relatively straightforward, it should be practiced to assure scope and patient safety. Understanding ultrasound physics helps users understand how changes in the acoustic interface alter imaging quality. Differentiation of echogenic structures, an understanding of color Doppler, and use of Gain, Depth, Measurement, and Frequency functions will help learners optimize ultrasound imaging, procedure performance. Knowing how to manipulate the image processor will help the learner train eventual assisting nursing staff.

Learning Objectives:

- The learner should be able to access the airway using the EBUS scope through an oral airway, an LMA, and an endotracheal tube.
- The learner should be able to alternate between white light and ultrasound views.
- The learner should be able to demonstrate use of the on/off, gain, depth, curser placement and nodal size measurement, frequency, and color Doppler controls on the image processor.

Guided Study Questions:

- How is echogenicity altered by acoustic properties of tissue media?
- How does frequency regulate penetration depth of the ultrasound beam?
- What are the principles of color Doppler?

References (in addition to those provided for this session)

- Nishina K, Hirooka K, Wiegand J, Dremel H. Principles and Practice of endoscopic ultrasound. In Bolliger CT et al (eds): Clinical Chest Ultrasound: From the ICU to the bronchoscopy suite. Prog Respir Res. Basel, Karger, 2009, vol 3, pp 110-127.

Didactics: Potential viewing of instructional video EBUS Physics: Principles and Terminology

Assessment Instruments: Image processor, needle and syringe 10-point Checklist

Part 3: Preparation

Monitors Required: Display panel

Other equipment required: EBUS Bronchoscopy station

EBUS box model with bifurcated airway and hypoechoic structures

Intubation head or Laerdal upper airway and torso model.

Time Duration

Set-up	10 minutes
Preparation	10 minutes
Simulation	10 minutes
Debrief	10-20 minutes

Part 4: Supporting Files (case scenario handouts)

Scenario # 1 (Airway access and image acquisition): A 70 year old male has slightly enlarged lymph nodes at the subcarinal (7) and lower right paratracheal stations (4R). He is referred for EBUS-TBNA for diagnosis.

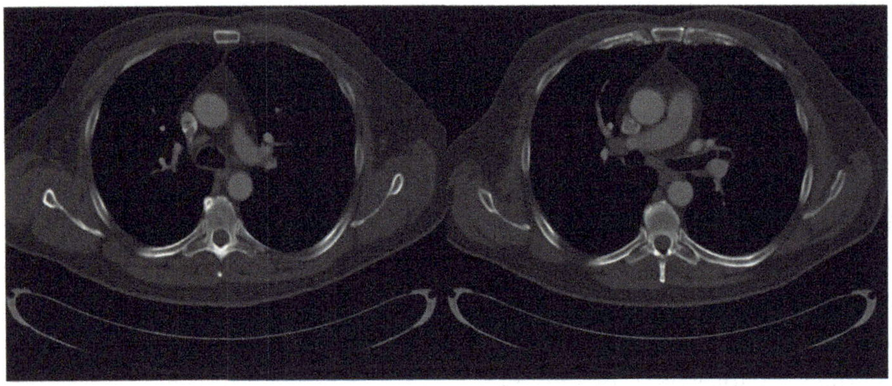

You must access the airway and demonstrate how to use the controls on the image processor in order to optimize image acquisition at these lymph node levels.

EBUS-TBNA Needle and Scope Handling

Case Information

Part 1: Demographics

Case Title: EBUS-TBNA of stations 7 and 4R
Subject Name: (1) Eddie Ebus
Scenario Name: EBUS-TBNA of stations 7 and 4R
Simulation Developer(s): H. Colt
Date(s) of Development: September 2022

Appropriate for following learning groups

Post graduate education, Physicians in practice
Specialties: Pulmonary, Anesthesiology, Surgery, Critical Care
Thoracic surgeons performing EBUS

Simulated patient 1 scenario

Scenario # 1 (10 minutes, with 10 minutes debriefing): With the EBUS bronchoscope in position inside the bifurcated airway model, the EBUS needle is used to puncture the lymph node visualized using EBUS.

Scenario description: The instructor will read the scenario to the team. It may be necessary for the instructor to demonstrate scope and needle handling techniques. The learner will then perform EBUS-TBNA of level 7 and 4R lymph node stations. The learner will articulate each step of needle handling, while another learner serves as the bronchoscopy assistant. It is assumed that approximately ten minutes per person will be devoted to the scenario, with 10 minutes for an instructor-led debriefing. The instructor may further choose to perform an additional ten minutes debriefing that includes viewing the EBUS curiosities instructional video.

* Template for Simulation Patient. Design Modified from original template by *Jeffrey M. Taekman, M.D, Duke University Simulation and Patient Safety Center*

Part 2: Curricular Information

Educational Rationale:

Learning to perform EBUS-TBNA using a step-by-step approach assures safe needle handling and acquisition of an adequate specimen without harming the bronchoscope or patient. Knowing how to manipulate the needle will additionally help the learner train assisting nursing staff.

Learning Objectives:

- The learner should be able to manipulate the EBUS scope and needle in the performance of EBUS-TBNA.
- The learner should be able to assist with EBUS-TBNA
- The learner should be able to demonstrate the various steps required for handling the scope, maintaining the ultrasound image, and handling the needle before, during and after EBUS-TBNA.

Guided Study Questions:

- Why does the needle sometimes not penetrate the lymph node?
- What alterations in balloon inflation and scope position might be necessary to optimize image acquisition?
- What precautions should be used during needle insertion and removal?

References (in addition to those provided for this session) NA

Didactics: Potential viewing of instructional video: EBUS Curiosities

Assessment Instruments: EBUS-STAT

Part 3: Preparation

Monitors Required: Display panel

Other equipment required: EBUS Bronchoscopy station

EBUS box model with bifurcated airway and hypoechoic structures

Time Duration

For this scenario

Set-up	10 minutes
Preparation	10 minutes
Simulation	10 minutes
Debrief	10-20 minutes

Part 4: Supporting Files (case scenario handouts)

Scenario # 1 (EBUS-TBNA): A 70-year old male has slightly enlarged lymph nodes at the subcarinal (7) and lower right paratracheal stations (4R). He is referred for EBUS-TBNA for diagnosis.

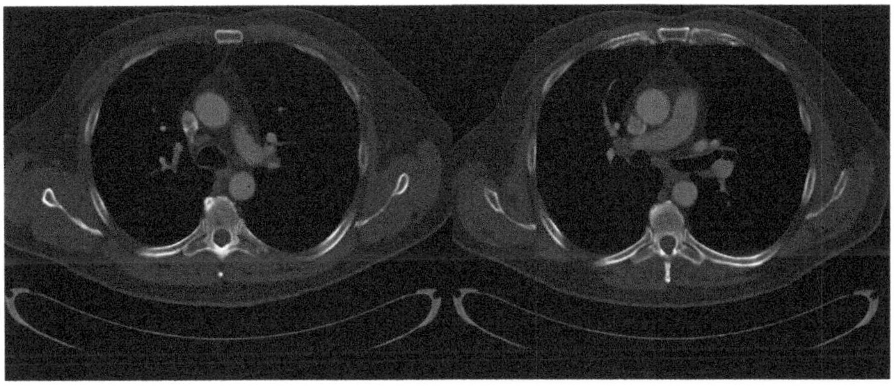

You must image the airway in order to visualize stations 4 and 7 after which you must perform EBUS-TBNA at levels 7 or 4R. One of the other participants will serve as your assistant. Please verbalize all needle and scope related commands.

****

SECTION 6

Observed Real-Patient Encounters

A series of *observed real-patient encounters* that include:

- An *informed consent, patient safety, procedural pause* encounter.
- An *EBUS-TBNA* image processor, needle and scope handling encounter.

* Checklists and assessment tools used at the discretion of program director.

USER INSTRUCTIONS

Real patient observations

The purpose of real patient observations is to allow the instructor to assess the learner in the clinical setting. This is similar to how medical students and other house officers are observed and judged prior to being deemed competent to perform a physical examination or certain procedures.

Various assessment tools and ten-point checklists are used to document knowledge and skill acquisition in accordance with elements required by ACGME (patient care, medical knowledge, practice-based learning and improvement, interpersonal communication skills, professionalism, and systems-based practice).

It is assumed that learners will be observed throughout their subspecialty training, and that specific instances may be chosen for assessment purposes. The frequency of such assessments is still undetermined, but the purpose is to be able to monitor the student's progression along the learning curve, so that instructors might be able to provide constructive feedback and advice, in addition to knowledge and technical expertise. These assessments can also be used for physicians in practice performing procedures under the guidance or observation of a proctor (certified trainer).

Learners are encouraged to build on the knowledge gained from simulation sessions, and to read (1) The psychological aspects of flexible bronchoscopy and informed consent process, (2) The extract from Institute for Clinical Systems Improvement Guidelines for Time Out (procedural pause), and (3) The extract from the Center for Disease Control's guide on Universal precautions.

The learner may wish to keep a diary of procedures performed. An example of such a log is provided below.

Patient identification	Date of procedure	Procedures performed EBUS-TBNA (and nodal stations sampled)	Complications (None if applicable)	Results (includes response to complications and laboratory data)
1				
2				
3				
4				
5				

EBUS and EBUS-TBNA Procedure log

Bronchoscopist ______________________________

Patient identification and Indication for procedure	Date of procedure	Procedures performed (EBUS-TBNA). Note nodal stations sampled	Complications (None if applicable)	Results (includes response to complications and laboratory data)
1				
2				
3				
4				
5				
6				
7				
8				
9				
10				
11				
12				
13				
14				
15				
16				
17				
18				
19				
20				
21				
22				
23				
24				
25				
26				
27				
28				
29				
30				

EBUS INFORMED CONSENT 10-Point CHECKLIST*

Learner ______________________ Training Year ______________

Faculty ______________________ Date ______________________

☐ Simulation EBUS-TBNA Workshop ☐ Patient-based EBUS-TBNA Scenario

Educational Item* Items 1-10 are scored 10 points each (no partial points given)	**Satisfactory Yes/No**
1. Able to define "Informed Consent": ☐ Informed decision-making regarding indications and expected outcomes, conflict of interest ☐ Protection from liability ☐ Provides opportunity to assess management strategies ☐ Provides opportunity to discuss risks, benefits, and alternatives	Yes / No
2. Able to discuss diagnosis and pertinent clinical issues	Yes / No
3. Able to describe the purpose of the procedure	Yes / No
4. Able to describe the nature of the procedure	Yes / No
5. Able to describe procedure-related risks	Yes / No
6. Able to describe procedure-related benefits	Yes / No
7. Able to describe alternative procedures regardless of cost or health care coverage	Yes / No
8. Able to describe potential risks and benefits from choosing the alternatives	Yes / No
9. Able to describe the risks and benefits of not performing the procedure or not choosing any of the alternatives	Yes / No
10. Able to demonstrate "effectiveness" of the informed consent process by asking the patient to explain in his or her own words, their understanding of the procedure	Yes / No

* Each of the 10 items contains all of the elements required by ACGME (patient care, medical knowledge, practice-based learning and improvement, interpersonal communication skills, professionalism, and systems-based practice).

FINAL GRADE PASS FAIL **SCORE** _______/100

EBUS PROCEDURAL PAUSE 10-Point CHECKLIST*

Learner ______________________________ Training Year ________________

Faculty ______________________________ Date ________________________

☐ Simulation EBUS Workshop ☐ Patient-based EBUS Scenario

Educational Item* Items 1-10 are scored 10 points each (no partial points given)	**Satisfactory Yes/No**
1. Able to define "Procedural Pause" as: ☐ Time-Out ☐ Wrong patient, site, procedure ☐ Team communication/patient understanding ☐ Mandatory in USA	Yes / No
2. Able to describe requirements of the procedural pause: ☐ Immediately before procedure ☐ Correct site, position, procedure ☐ Correct patient ☐ Pertinent medical records and equipment ☐ Verbal acknowledgements by all team members ☐ Elimination of environmental distractions	Yes / No
3. Able to describe the team leader's role	Yes / No
4. Able to describe the nursing team's role	Yes / No
5. Able to describe the patient's role	Yes / No
6. Able to describe other person's roles (technicians, other physicians)	Yes / No
7. Able to list the elements that must be covered: ☐ Patient ☐ Procedure ☐ Side and site ☐ Informed consent ☐ Medical records and equipment ☐ Medications ☐ Allergies/drug reactions ☐ Safety concerns based on history	Yes / No
8. Able to address behaviors in case of distractions	Yes / No
9. Able to describe behaviors in case of disagreements	Yes / No
10. Able to describe other elements pertaining to assuring a culture of safety: ☐ Communication ☐ Ability to prevent and respond to complications ☐ Universal, Droplet, and Airborne pathogen precautions	Yes / No

*Each of the 10 items contains all of the elements required by ACGME (patient care, medical knowledge, practice-based learning and improvement, interpersonal communication skills, professionalism, and systems-based practice).

FINAL GRADE PASS FAIL **SCORE** _______/100

EBUS Image Processor, Needle and Scope Handling 10-Point CHECKLIST*

Learner ______________________ Training Year ______________

Faculty ______________________ Date ______________

☐ Interactive session ☐ Patient environment

Educational Item* Items 1-10 are scored 10 points each (**no partial points given**)	**Satisfactory Yes/No**
1. Airway access and alternate among EBUS and White light bronchoscopy ☐ Airway access Oral/LMA/ET Tube ☐ Alternate EBUS/WLB	Yes / No
2. Image quality adjustments: **Depth** ☐ Describe ☐ Demonstrate	Yes / No
3. Image quality adjustments: **Gain** ☐ Describe ☐ Demonstrate	Yes / No
4. Image quality adjustments: **Frequency** ☐ Describe ☐ Demonstrate	Yes / No
5. Image quality adjustments: **Doppler** ☐ Describe ☐ Demonstrate	Yes / No
6. Image target measurements: **Cursor placement** ☐ Able to describe cursor placement for measuring lymph node size ☐ Able to demonstrate cursor placement and size measurements	Yes / No
7. Scope: Able to demonstrate balloon placement and functionality for optimal image acquisition ☐ Balloon placement onto scope ☐ Balloon integrity check ☐ Removal of air bubbles	Yes / No
8. Needle: Able to check mechanics and integrity of: ☐ Needle adjuster lock ☐ sheath adjuster knob ☐ Connecting slide	Yes / No
9. Needle: Integrity, retraction, and slider ☐ Integrity ☐ Retracts into sheath ☐ Slider moves freely and locks	Yes / No
10. Needle: Stylet and aspiration syringe integrity and function ☐ Moves freely ☐ Aspiration syringe functions	Yes / No

* Each of the 10 items contains all of the elements required by ACGME (patient care, medical knowledge, practice-based learning and improvement, interpersonal communication skills, professionalism, and systems-based practice).

FINAL GRADE PASS FAIL **SCORE** _______/100

SECTION 7

Practical Approach Sessions

Interactive Patient-centered
Practical Approach to Procedural Decision-making exercises

USER INSTRUCTIONS

Practical Approach Workshops

The purpose of these practical approach sessions is to help learners think through the decision-making process. Often, instructors will use a practical approach to help students gain insights into the strategy and planning, technical performance, and response to complications elements of a minimally invasive procedure.

These exercises are done orally, and the assessment is subjective, based on the instructor's perception of how the learner responds to questions and outlines a procedural strategy. Learners are taught to use scientific evidence as well as expert opinion to formulate plans and achieve desired results. A dialogue is thus engendered between instructor and student in order to address alternatives and differences in technique, as well as expected outcomes.

It is expected that sessions last no more than 30 minutes. The learner may be given a scenario, and using a model of the four-box approach the learner might be asked to address each of the four boxes, with specific emphasis on one or two items based on instructor preference. Numerous exercises are available on the Bronchoscopy.org website, but any scenario the instructor creates can be used for teaching purposes.

Four Box Approach

Initial Evaluation	**Procedural Strategies and planning**
1. Physical examination, complementary tests, and functional status assessment 2. Patient's significant comorbidities 3. Patient's support system (also includes family) 4. Patient preferences and expectations (also includes family)	1. Indications, contraindications, and expected results 2. Operator and team experience and expertise 3. Risk-benefits analysis and therapeutic alternatives 4. Respect for persons (Informed Consent and ethics issues)
Procedural Techniques and results	**Long term Management Plan**
1. Anesthesia and other perioperative care 2. Techniques and instrumentation 3. Anatomic dangers and other risks 4. Results and procedure-related complications	1. Outcome assessment 2. Follow-up tests, visits, and procedures 3. Referrals to medical, surgical, or palliative/end of life subspecialty care 4. Quality improvement and team evaluation of clinical encounter

The Patient-centered practical approach is an interactive learning program:

- The purpose of *The Practical Approach* is to help learners gain the cognitive, technical, experiential, and affective skills necessary to perform bronchoscopy. Competency is sought in the three major elements of a procedure; strategy and planning, execution, and response to procedure-related adverse events or complications.
- Using a four-box approach inspired from Albert Jonsen's[1] classic work in medical ethics, learners rationalize various components of the decision-making process.
  - By working through case scenarios, learners are prompted to think about the how and why of their actions, based on background information, pertinent literature, and experience.
  - Consistent with the ACGME professionalism competency guides[2,3], case scenarios prompt learners to address various components of the informed consent process, and discuss outcomes based on possible as well as real results.
- *The Practical Approach* helps learners become competent bronchoscopists according to current recommendations set forth by the American College of Graduate Medical Education[4] whereby trainees learn to:
  - Gather essential and accurate information about their patients.
  - Make informed decisions about diagnostic and therapeutic interventions based on patient information and preferences, up-to-date scientific evidence and clinical judgment.
  - Use information technology to support patient care decisions and patient education.
  - Develop patient management plans.
  - Counsel and educate patients and their families.
  - Communicate effectively and demonstrate caring and respectful behaviors when interacting with patients and their families.
  - Provide healthcare services aimed at preventing health problems or maintaining health.
  - Work with healthcare professionals, including those from other disciplines to provide patient-focused care.

References

1. Jonsen AR, Siegler M, Winslade WJ. Clinical Ethics. 6th Ed, McGraw Hill, NY 2006.
2. ACGME Web site:http//www.acgme.org/outcome/comp/compfull.asp
3. Apelgren K. ACGME e-Bulletin. August 2006
4. ACGME Competencies at http://www.acgme.org
5. *Patient-centered approach to central airways disorders.* Colt HG and Murgu S, Published, Elsevier Press 2012.

Practical Approach Module

EBUS-TBNA for lymph nodes < 1 cm in a patient with solitary pulmonary nodule

Based on the information below, please describe your procedural decision making and answer the three questions at the end of the exercise. Do your best to complete each item of the Four Boxes. If the case scenario contains no information pertaining to an item, please address it as NOT AVAILABLE. Each case scenario may have greater emphasis on one or more items listed.

This 55-year-old man has a 1.5 cm solitary pulmonary nodule in the mediobasal segment of right lower lobe which was incidentally noted while he was undergoing CT of the abdomen for nephrolithiasis. The scan shows a 1.5 cm RLL nodule, 5.5 SUV on PET and a 7 mm subcarinal lymph node on CT which is not PET-avid. He has no risk factors for cancer. Vital signs are normal. Physical exam is unremarkable. CBC, coagulation and chemistry panel, and spirometry are normal. PPD is negative. He is an attorney specializing in real estate law. He lives with his wife and 1 child. He has no advanced directives. He desires treatment in case of lung cancer.

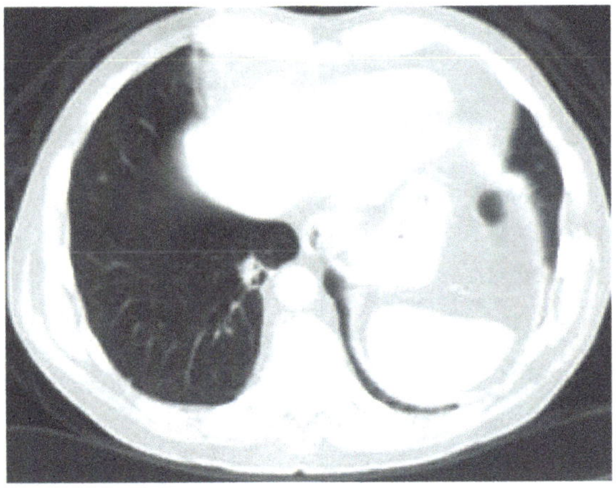

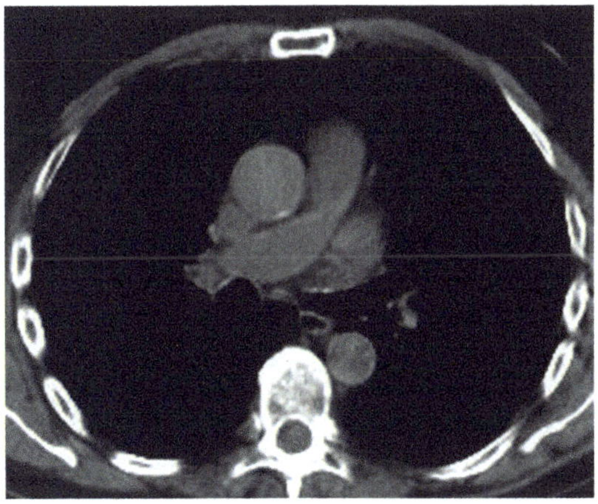

After addressing items of the four boxes, please consider the following:

- Describe major elements of informed consent.
- Describe the current evidence about staging CT/PET negative mediastinal lymphadenopathy in patients with known or suspected lung cancer.
- List three reasons for a poor sample on smear.

Initial Evaluation	**Procedural Strategies and planning**
1. Physical examination, complementary tests, and functional status assessment 2. Patient's significant comorbidities 3. Patient's support system (also includes family) 4. Patient preferences and expectations (also includes family)	1. Indications, contraindications, and expected results 2. Operator and team experience and expertise 3. Risk-benefits analysis and therapeutic alternatives 4. Respect for persons (Informed Consent and ethics issues)
Procedural Techniques and results	**Long term Management Plan**
1. Anesthesia and other perioperative care 2. Techniques and instrumentation 3. Anatomic dangers and other risks 4. Results and procedure-related complications	1. Outcome assessment 2. Follow-up tests, visits, and procedures 3. Referrals to medical, surgical, or palliative/end of life subspecialty care 4. Quality improvement and team evaluation of clinical encounter

Practical Approach b&w

EBUS-TBNA for lymph nodes < 1 cm in a patient with known solitary pulmonary nodule

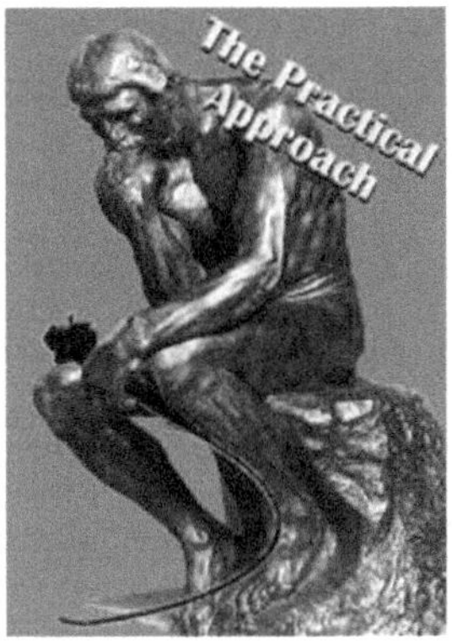

- Describe major elements of informed consent.
- Describe the current debate about staging CT/PET negative mediastinal lymphadenopathy in patients with known or suspected lung cancer.
- List three reasons for a poor sample on smear.

www.Bronchoscopy.org

Case description

- 55-year-old man with 1.5 cm solitary pulmonary nodule in the mediobasalsegment of right lower lobe which was incidentally noted while he was undergoing CT of abdomen for nephrolithiasis. He has no risk factors for cancer. Vital signs are normal. Physical exam is unremarkable. CBC, coagulation and chemistry panel, and spirometry are normal. PPD is negative. He is an attorney specializing in real estate law. He lives with his wife and 1 child. He has no advanced directives. He desires all available treatment options in case he has lung cancer.

www.Bronchoscopy.org

Initial Evaluation

- Good performance status
- Excellent and supportive support system
- History of Nephrolithiasis
- Desires diagnosis and treatment
- 1.5 cm RLL spn, 5.5 SUV on PET
- 7 mm subcarinal lymph node on CT which is not PET avid

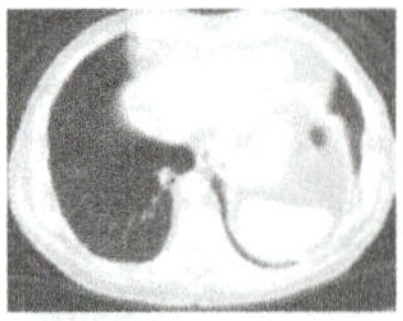

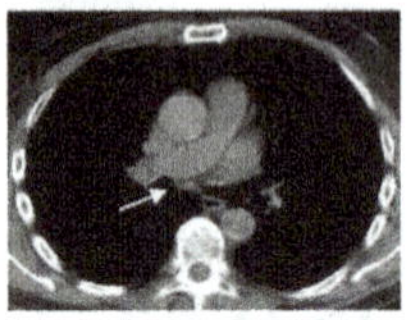

www.Bronchoscopy.org

Procedural Strategies

- Indications
  - Invasive lymph node staging in a patient withradiographically (CT and PET) normal mediastinum
  - PET scan and Integrated PET/CT have demonstrated ahigh NPV for mediastinal nodal disease with NPV of~90%*
  - 5.6% of patients with radiographically stage 1 disease were found to have N2 disease** ■ Risk factors and incidence of occult N2 mets include***
    - **larger tumor size (≥6.0 cm) –57% prevalence**
    - **central location-21.6% prevalence**
    - **high PET SUV (≥4.0)-10.5% prevalence**
    - **adeno ca cell type-9.0% prevalence**

*Eur Respir J 2009; 33: 201–212

***J Thorac Cardiovasc Surg*2006;131:822-829

****Ann Thorac Surg 2007;84:177-18*

www.Bronchoscopy.org

Procedural Strategies

- Indications
  - Should this patient undergo lymph node stagingbefore or after needle aspiration biopsy of hisperipheral nodule?
  - Should he undergo invasive lymph node staging?
    - Invasive staging should be reserved for patients with 1or more risk factors for occult N2 disease* ** ***
    - Routine use of invasive lymph node staging for patientswith clinical stage 1 non small cell lung ca and no riskfactors for occult N2 disease is not cost effective**

**Ann ThoracSurg2007;84:177-181*

*** J ThoracCardiovascSurg2006;131:822-829*

**** EurJ CardiothoracSurg. 2007 Jul;32(1):1-8*

www.Bronchoscopy.org

Procedural Strategies

- Contraindications:
  - None
- Expected Results:
  - EBUS-TBNA demonstrated 89% sensitivity, 100%specificity, 98.9% NPV for 5-10 mm radio graphicallynormal nodes*
- Operator and team experience: well experienced team
- Risks-benefits:
  - Safe procedure with no serious complicationsreported in the literature.
  - Agitation, cough, and presence of blood at puncturesite have been reported as infrequentcomplications.**
  - Benefits: highly accurate and safe procedure toobtain tissue for staging. Same day procedure

**Chest 2008;133;887-891*

**Eur Respir J 2009; 33: 1156–1164

www.Bronchoscopy.org

Procedural Strategies

- Diagnostic alternatives:
  - Transbronchial needle aspiration
    - Sensitivity 65-89% for subcarinal node location > 1cm*
    - Sensitivity 39% if median prevalence of disease is 34%**
    - High false negative rate 28%*** requires negative results to be followed with another invasive staging procedure
    - Histology needles provide increased diagnostic yield except when lesions are <1 cm*
    - In a head to head comparison sensitivity/NPV was 36%/78% and 69%/88% for TBNA vsEBUS-TBNA respectively****
    - A therapeutic strategy using both TBNA and EBUS TBNA**** or TBNA and EUS-FNA *****has been proposed as the most cost effective strategy for staging the mediastinum

***Am J RespirCritCare Med* 2000;161:601–607

**Thorax 2005;60:949–955

****Chest 2007;132;202-220*

*****JAMA. 2008;299(5):540-546*

*****J Bronchol2008;15:17–20

****** Lung Cancer 64 (2009) 127–128

www.Bronchoscopy.org

Procedural Strategies

- Risks-Benefits
  - Cost effectiveness-no formal evaluations have been published
    - In 2 separate decision-analytic models, both (EUS-FNA + EBUS-FNA) and (conventional TBNA + EBUS-FNA) were more cost-effective approaches than mediastinoscopy for staging patients with NSCLC and abnormal mediastinal lymph nodes on non-invasive imaging* **
    - A strategy adding EUS-FNA to a conventional lung ca staging approach (mediastinoscopy & thoracotomy) reduced costs by 40% per patient***
    - May actually increase health care costs if done in low volume centers by less experienced operators**** *****
  - Start up costs (as of 2011-2012)
    - Cost of equipment ~100K******and training
    - Physician reimbursement ~$280; facility reimbursement $257******

*Gastrointestinal Endoscopy 69, No. 2, Supp 1, 2009, S260

**J Bronchol2008;15:17–20

****Thorax 2004;59;596-601*

*****Lung Cancer 64 (2009) 127–128*

*****J Bronchol2008; 15:127-128

****** *Southern Medical Journal 2008;101,No5;534-38*

www.Bronchoscopy.org

Procedural Strategies

- Diagnostic alternatives:
  - Percutaneous needle aspiration of nodule
  - Endoscopic ultrasound in a head to head comparison* sensitivity and negative predictive value (69% and 89% respectively) was identical to EBUS for accessible nodes
  - Mediastinoscopy gold standard.
    - Mediastinoscopy is invasive staging procedure of choice in radiographicallynegative mediastinum** ***
      - 42% sensitivity in clinical stage 1 ****
      - Difficult to access level 7 nodes
  - VATS most invasive of alternatives. Only provides access to ipsilateral nodes. 75% sensitivity****. Benefits include definitive lobar resection at same time if node negative.

*JAMA. 2008;299(5):540-546

**Chest 2007;132;178S-201S*

***EurJ CardiothoracSurg. 2007 Jul;32(1):1-8

****Chest 2007;132;202-220

www.Bronchoscopy.org

Procedural Strategies

- Informed consent:
  - There were no barriers to learning identified. Patient has good insight into his disease and realistic expectations.

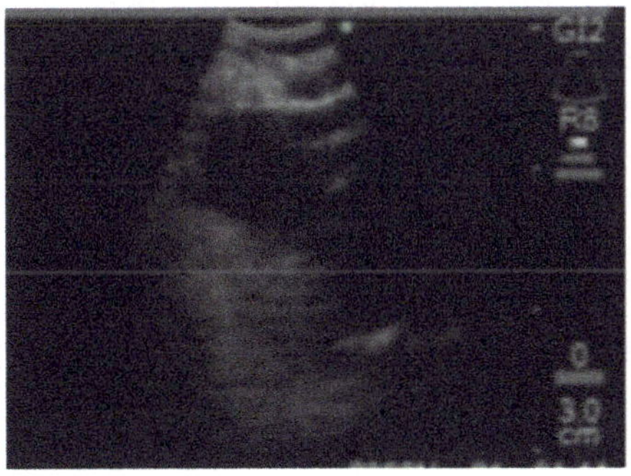

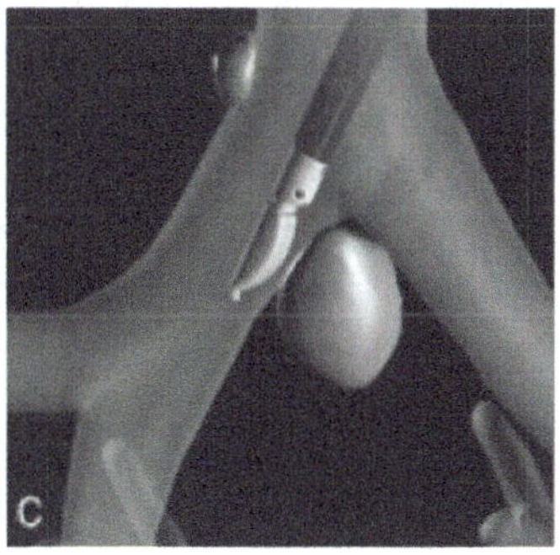

Drawing from HerthFJ et al. Chest 2003;123:604 –7

EBUS image from patient.

www.Bronchoscopy.org

Procedural techniques and results Anesthesia and perioperative care

- Conscious sedation
  - May be performed in bronchoscopy suite
  - Cost savings compared to general anesthesia.
  - Visualization and biopsy of smaller nodes technically more difficult than with general anesthesia.
- General anesthesia with LMA
  - Better visualization of higher nodes compared with ET tube
  - May be performed in bronchoscopy suite
  - May not be appropriate in severe obesity or severe untreated GERD
- General anesthesia with ET tube
  - Usually performed in OR
  - EBUS scope directed more centrally in airway which may make biopsies more difficult

BI #. Practical Approach Title

Procedural techniques and results: Moderate Sedation or General Anesthesia?

- As more and more centers begin EBUS-TBNA programs, it is important that the procedure is performed in the correct environment and with realistic expectations of patients, operators, and equipment performance characteristics.
- If a consensus is reached that complete nodal staging is feasible and accurate with EBUS-TBNA, it may be more optimally performed under general anesthesia until the bronchoscopist feels comfortable in targeting these smaller lymph nodes in multiple stations in a conscious patient.

Chest 2008;134;1350-1351

Procedural Techniques and Results

- Instrumentation
  - EBUS scope-direct real time US imaging with curved array ultrasound transducer incorporated in distal end of bronchoscope
  - Ultrasound processor
    - Adjustable gain and depth
    - B mode and Doppler capabilities
  - Needle
    - 22 gauge acrogenic needle with stylet
    - Needle guide system locks to scope
    - Lockable needle and sheath
    - Precise needle projection up to 4 cm

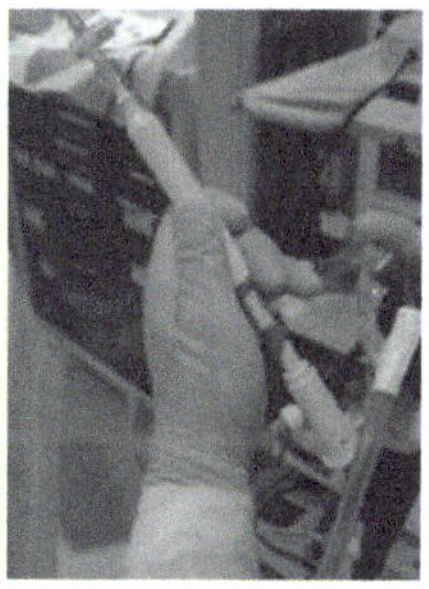

www.Bronchoscopy.org

Procedural Techniques and Results

- Anatomic dangers and other risks
  - Major blood vessels-azygous, PA, aorta, SVC and Left atrium
    - Risk of canulating major vessel significantly reduced with real time B mode and Doppler mode imaging
    - "Minor" oozing of blood at puncture site was reported in 1 study. There have been no reports of major bleeding*
  - Pneumothorax and pneumomediastinum**
    - Have been reported with blind TBNA but no reports in literature with EBUS guided FNA.
  - A case of bacterial pericardial effusion and nodal infection have recently been reported as complications following EBUS with full needle extension***.

www.Bronchoscopy.org

Procedural Techniques and Results

- Aspirate cytology
  - Adequate/representative in presence of frankly malignant cells, lymphocytes, lymphoid tissue, or clusters of anthracotic pigment-laden macrophages*
  - Inadequate/nonrepresentative if there are no cellular components, scant lymphocytes (defined as <40 per HPF) blood only, or cartilage or bronchial epithelial cells only* **
  - A quantitative cut off value of at least 30% of cellularity composed of lymphocytes has been arbitrarily proposed by some experts***
  - Higher yield may be obtained by obtaining aspirates from the periphery of nodes****

**Am J Clin Pathol* 2008;130:434-443

***Chest* 2008;134;368-374;

****Chest* 2004;126;1005-1006

*****Techniques in GI Endoscopy*, Vol 2, No 3, 2000. pp 136-141

www.Bronchoscopy.org

Procedural Techniques and Results

- Number of aspirates* if ROSE not utilized
  - Best yield with 3 aspirates per station (see table)
  - Two aspirations per LN station can be acceptable when at least one tissue core specimen is obtained by the first two aspirations
    - Sensitivity 91.7%, NPV 96.0%, and accuracy 97.2%
  - If operator believes targeting is inadequate or insufficient another aspirate should be performed

	Aspirations, No.			
Variables	**1**	**2**	**3**	**4**
Sensitivity	69.8 (30/43)	83.7 (36/43)	95.3 (41/43)	95.3 (41/43)
Specificity	100 (83/83)	100 (83/83)	100 (83/83)	100 (83/83)
PPV	100 (30/30)	100 (36/36)	100 (41/41)	100 (41/41)
NPV	86.5 (83/96)	92.2 (83/90)	97.6 (83/85)	97.6 (83/85)
Accuracy	89.7 (113/126)	94.4 (119/126)	98.4 (124/126)	98.4 (124/126)

* Data are presented as % (No./total). We considered inadequate samples as negative results.

BI #. Practical Approach Title

* Chest 2008;134;368-374;

www.Bronchoscopy.org

Maximum results after 3 aspirates

Table 2 – Cumulatice Diagnostic Values of EBUS-TBNA Shown by the Number of Aspirations*

	Aspirations, No.			
Variables	**1**	**2**	**3**	**4**
Sensitivity	69.8 (30/43)	83.7 (36/43)	95.3 (41/43)	95.3 (41/43)
Specificity	100 (83/83)	100 (83/83)	100 (83/83)	100 (83/83)
PPV	100 (30/30)	100 (36/36)	100 (41/41)	100 (41/41)
NPV	86.5 (83/96)	92.2 (83/90)	97.6 (83/85)	97.6 (83/85)
Accuracy	89.7 (113/126)	94.4 (119/126)	98.4 (124/126)	98.4 (124/126)

* Data are presented as % (No./total). We considered inadequate samples as negative results.

Sample adequacy reached 100% in three aspirations. Median procedure time was 1 h when three nodal stations were punctured. Results suggest that a fourth aspiration is not necessary in EBUS-TBNA for the mediastinal staging of NSCLC. The sensitivity of the first aspiration was 68.9%. The sensitivity increased to 83.7% after two aspirations and to 95.3% after three aspirations.

Chest 2008;134;368-37417

www.Bronchoscopy.org

Procedural Techniques and Results

- Results and procedure-related complications
  - Due to the absence of history suggestive of a non-cancer diagnosis and high SUV on PET, the level 7 node was sampled using EBUS under general anesthesia and a 9.0 endotracheal tube.
  - The cytology was diagnostic for non small cell carcinoma (adenocarcinoma).
  - There were no complications.

www.Bronchoscopy.org

Long-term Management Plan

- Outcome assessment
  - Patient was referred for multidisciplinary evaluation to include cardiothoracic surgery, oncology, and radiation oncology for potential trial enrollment for neoadjuvant treatment of stage IIIA adenocarcinoma of the lung.*
- Follow-up tests and procedures
  - Patient will follow up in 1 month to ensure he has been evaluated by all the above specialties.
- Referrals
  - See above.
- Quality improvement
  - The occult N2 metastasis was identified prior to the patient undergoing VATS or open thoracotomy for a non resectable tumor.
  - 5 year survival for IIIA non-small cell lung ca is 23%.

**Chest 2007;132;243S-265S*

www.Bronchoscopy.org

Question 1: Major elements of informed consent

- Protects the patient by providing them with complete information on which to make an informed decision.
- Protects the health care provider from liability provided the procedure is properly executed according to the prevailing standards of care in the community and without negligence.
- Gives the health care providers an opportunity to consider and re-consider the diagnostic and therapeutic strategies being proposed
- Allows for a discussion of possible risks and benefits and to prepare for procedure-related events.

www.Bronchoscopy.org

From a legal standpoint, consent for a medical procedure must be both informed and effective

To be *informed*, a patient must be given information about the procedure relevant to their individual situation.

To be *effective*, the person undergoing the procedure should be able to demonstrate, in his or her own words, their understanding of the procedure or treatment.

www.Bronchoscopy.org

American Medical Association: Informed consent is a *process* which should disclose and discuss:

- The patient's diagnosis and concerning clinical issues.
- The nature and purpose of the proposed procedure
- The risks and benefits of the proposed procedure.
- Alternative regardless of cost or coverage by health insurance.
- Potential risks and benefits from choosing the alternatives.
- The risks and benefits of <u>not</u> receiving or undergoing treatment or procedures.

Question 2: Describe debate about staging CT/PET negative mediastinal lymphadenopathy

- PET scan and Integrated PET/CT have demonstrated a high NPV for mediastinal nodal disease with NPV of ~90%.
- 5.6% of patients with radiographically stage 1 disease have N2 disease.
- Risk factors and incidence of occult N2 disease:
  - **larger tumor size (≥6.0 cm) – 57% prevalence**
  - **central location- 21.6% prevalence**
  - **high PET SUV (≥4.0)- 10.5% prevalence**
  - **adeno ca cell type- 9.0% prevalence**

Indications for nodal staging in CT/PET negative patients

- Should these patients undergo invasive lymph node staging?
  - Invasive staging should probably be reserved for patients with 1 or more risk factors for occult N2 disease.
  - Routine use of invasive lymph node staging for patients with clinical stage 1 non small cell lung ca and no risk factors for occult N2 disease is probably not cost effective.
  - While others propose that all nodes be sampled (especially in view of new developments pertaining to tumor markers)

Furthermore

- Adenocarcinoma is a frequent histologic type of NSCLC. Data suggest that patients with adenocarcinoma (contrary to squamous cell carcinoma) may have false negative PET/CT findings of the mediastinum
- This suggests that adenocarcinoma should probably be carefully staged preoperatively even in mediastinal PET/CT-negative cases.

Chest; Prepublished online December 31, 2008;

www.Bronchoscopy.org

EBUS for PET negative, normal mediastinum

- Patients highly suspicious for NSCLC with CT scans showing no enlarged lymph nodes (no node > 1 cm) and a negative PET finding of the mediastinum underwent EBUS- TBNA.
- Identifiable lymph nodes at locations 2R, 2L, 4R, 4L, 7, 10R, 10L, 11R, and 11L were aspirated.
- All patients underwent subsequent surgical staging. Diagnoses based on aspiration results were compared with those based on surgical results.
- One hundred patients (mean age, 52.4 years; 59 men) were included. After surgery, 97 patients (mean age, 52.9 years; 57 men) had NSCLC confirmed and were included in the analysis.

Herth F et al. CHEST 2008; 133:887–891

www.Bronchoscopy.org

- In this group, 156 lymph nodes ranging 5 to 10 mm in size were detected and sampled.
  - **Malignancy was detected in nine patients** but missed in one patient.
  - Mean diameter of the punctured lymph nodes was 7.9 mm.
  - The sensitivity of EBUS-TBNA for detecting malignancy was 89%, specificity was 100%, and the negative predictive value was 98.9%. No complications occurred.
- EBUS-TBNA can be used to accurately sample and stage patients with clinical stage 1 lung cancer and no evidence of mediastinal involvement on CT and PET.
- Potentially operable patients with no signs of mediastinal involvement may benefit from presurgical staging with EBUS-TBNA.

Herth F et al. CHEST 2008; 133:887–891

www.Bronchoscopy.org

Table 1: ***All Patients With Confirmed Mediastinal Involvement*** *

Patient No.	Lymph Node Station	Node Stage	Histology	Local Primary	Size Primary, cm
1	10r	N1	Squamous	RLL	2.4
2	7	N2	Adeno	LUL	2.8
3	4r	N2	Adeno	RUL	1.5
4	7	N2	Adeno	RLL	3.2
5	10r	N1	Adeno	RLL	2.8
6	4r	N2	Adeno	LUL	2.2
7	4r	N3	Adeno	LLL	2.7
8	7r	N2	Adeno	RUL	3.0
9†	10r	N1	Adeno	RLL	2.5

*RUL = right upper lobe; RLL right lower lobe; LUL = left upper lobe; LLL = left lower lobe; Adeno = adenocarcinoma.

† Missed by EBUS-TBNA.

Herth F et al. CHEST 2008; 133:887–891

www.Bronchoscopy.org

The size of PET-negative nodes also impact probability of malignancy

Mediastinal lymph nodes and relation with metastatic involvement: a metanalysis
Langen et al, Eur J Cardiothorac Surg 2006;29:26-29

- Probability for malignancy in lymph nodes measuring 10- 15 mm in the short axis is 29%,and about 60% if nodes are larger.
- **If nodes 10-15 mm and PET Negative**, probability for malignancy is 5%. (1 of 20 nodes) Perhaps Refrain from mediastinoscopy
- **If nodes > 16 mm and PET Negative**, probability for malignancy is 21%, (1 of 5 nodes)
  - Perhaps Proceed with mediastinoscopy

Lymph node size category	NPV (%)	PPV (%)
CT 10–15 mm	95	62
CT 16–20mm	81	90
CT >20 mm, with outlier	82	90
CT >20 mm, without outlier	80	90

www.Bronchoscopy.org

Question 3: Reasons for poor sampling and smears From G. Marcielli, with permission

- Sample coagulation : delay in processing may completely hinder process of smearing on the slide because of coagulation, even when blood content of the sample is not too much. Sample coagulation occurs in the needle lumen or on the slide surface.
- Air drying artefacts : if Papanicolaou (fig. A&B) stain is required, the smear must be wet when fixative is applied, otherwise staining artefacts are the rule. Conversely, with Diff-Quick stain, the quantity of sample fluid must be just enough to smear, enabling the sample to dry as soon as possible.
- Air bubbles : their presence in the material put on the slide causes uneven smear distribution.
- Thick smear : the correct technique provides distribution of cells in monolayer on slide surface; cells overlapping makes the examination of precise cellular details difficult or impossible To avoid this problem smear only a **small** drop of sample on the slide surface.
- Crushed smear : results from excessive pressure applied to smea3r0 the sample; this may completely destroy diagnostic material.

www.Bronchoscopy.org

SECTION 8

Proctored EBUS & EBUS-TBNA

Proctored patient-care in the procedural setting

USER INSTRUCTIONS

Proctored EBUS and EBUS-TBNA

The purpose of proctoring a procedure is to document that a physician is indeed able to independently perform all the elements of EBUS & EBUS-TBNA. These include strategy and planning, technique, patient safety measures and the ability to respond appropriately to procedure-related adverse events.

The Proctored EBUS-TBNA ten-point assessment tool can be used for grading purposes. This tool summarizes information contained in the Informed Consent, Procedural Pause, Practical Approach, and Sedation/Anesthesia checklists, as well as items contained in the Processor-Needle-Syringe checklist and EBUS-STAT assessment tool.

The overall assessment should also include the faculty's general observations of the learner's practices during the course of training. From an assessment perspective, this is the last item with which to "assess" a learner's ability to competently perform EBUS bronchoscopy. The intensity with which proctoring occurs, and the number of "proctored" cases that may be required within a training program or health care institution for physicians in-practice is variable.

EBUS PROCTORED EBUS & EBUS-TBNA 10-Point CHECKLIST*

Learner ______________________________ Training Year ________________

Faculty ______________________________ Date ________________________

☐ Simulation EBUS Workshop ☐ Patient-based EBUS Scenario

Educational Item* Items 1-10 are scored 10 points each (no partial points given)	**Satisfactory Yes/No**
1. Formulation of effective plan and strategy: ☐ Informed consent obtained, signed and in medical record ☐ History and physical ☐ Review imaging studies ☐ Cost-effective practice ☐ Use of information resources ☐ Applies evidence-based medicine ☐ Use of systems resources	Yes / No
2. Patient safety: ☐ ASA assessment ☐ Airway assessment ☐ Allergies ☐ Medications ☐ Comorbidities	Yes / No
3. Patient safety: ☐ Positioning ☐ Supplemental oxygen ☐ Vital signs ☐ Suction ☐ Bite-block and/or ET tube if applicable ☐ Verifies ability to respond to complications and accessibility of resuscitation equipment	Yes / No
4. Patient and procedural team safety: ☐ Knowledgeable use of image processor ☐ Hand disinfection ☐ Universal precautions ☐ "Time-Out".	Yes / No
5. Procedure: ☐ Premedication ☐ Moderate sedation ☐ Topical anesthetic ☐ General anesthesia as applicable	Yes / No
6. Procedure: ☐ Scope insertion ☐ Empathy and Communication with patient	Yes / No
7. Procedure: ☐ Image processor controls ☐ Balloon attachment and troubleshooting ☐ Needle, stylet, and syringe function and troubleshooting	Yes / No
8. Procedure: ☐ Alternate between white light and EBUS ☐ Image acquisition ☐ Recognition of mediastinal and hilar nodal anatomy ☐ Recognition of mediastinal and hilar vascular structures ☐ Lymph node sampling ☐ Smear preparation and station labeling	Yes / No
9. Communication with staff, patient, and patient family ☐ Puts needs of patient first ☐ Punctuality ☐ Respect ☐ Listening skills ☐ Personal appearance ☐ Initiative & ☐ Motivation ☐ Empathy ☐ Honesty ☐ Accepts responsibility	Yes / No
10. Documentation/procedure note ☐ Informative ☐ Accurate ☐ Communication with colleagues	Yes / No

* Contains elements required by ACGME (patient care, medical knowledge, practice-based learning and improvement, interpersonal communication skills, professionalism, and systems-based practice).

FINAL GRADE PASS FAIL **SCORE** _______/100

EBUS PROCTORED EBUS & EBUS-TBNA 10-Point CHECKLIST*

Learner ______________________ Training Year ______________

Faculty ______________________ Date ______________________

☐ Simulation EBUS Workshop ☐ Patient-based EBUS Scenario

Educational Item* Items 1-10 are scored 10 points each (no partial points given)	**Satisfactory Yes/No**
1. Formulation of effective plan and strategy: ☐ Informed consent obtained, signed and in medical record ☐ History and physical ☐ Review imaging studies ☐ Cost-effective practice ☐ Use of information resources ☐ Applies evidence-based medicine ☐ Use of systems resources	Yes / No
2. Patient safety: ☐ ASA assessment ☐ Airway assessment ☐ Allergies ☐ Medications ☐ Comorbidities	Yes / No
3. Patient safety: ☐ Positioning ☐ Supplemental oxygen ☐ Vital signs ☐ Suction ☐ Bite-block and/or ET tube if applicable ☐ Verifies ability to respond to complications and accessibility of resuscitation equipment	Yes / No
4. Patient and procedural team safety: ☐ Knowledgeable use of image processor ☐ Hand disinfection ☐ Universal precautions ☐ "Time-Out".	Yes / No
5. Procedure: ☐ Premedication ☐ Moderate sedation ☐ Topical anesthetic ☐ General anesthesia as applicable	Yes / No
6. Procedure: ☐ Scope insertion ☐ Empathy and Communication with patient	Yes / No
7. Procedure: ☐ Image processor controls ☐ Balloon attachment and troubleshooting ☐ Needle, stylet, and syringe function and troubleshooting	Yes / No
8. Procedure: ☐ Alternate between white light and EBUS ☐ Image acquisition ☐ Recognition of mediastinal and hilar nodal anatomy ☐ Recognition of mediastinal and hilar vascular structures ☐ Lymph node sampling ☐ Smear preparation and station labeling	Yes / No
9. Communication with staff, patient, and patient family ☐ Puts needs of patient first ☐ Punctuality ☐ Respect ☐ Listening skills ☐ Personal appearance ☐ Initiative & Motivation ☐ Empathy ☐ Honesty ☐ Accepts responsibility	Yes / No
10. Documentation/procedure note ☐ Informative ☐ Accurate ☐ Communication with colleagues	Yes / No

* Each of the 10 items contains all of the elements required by ACGME (patient care, medical knowledge, practice-based learning and improvement, interpersonal communication skills, professionalism, and systems-based practice).

FINAL GRADE PASS FAIL **SCORE** _______/100

SECTION 9

Assessment Tools*

A collection of assessment tools and user instructions:

- EBUS-STAT
- EBUS-SAT
- Post test of the Essential EBUS Bronchoscopist

**All assessment tools, including post-tests for The Essential EBUS Bronchoscopist and EBUS-STAT quiz can be found in a separate appendix.*

Scoring Recommendations for EBUS Assessment Tools

The goal of these assessment tools is to be able to monitor a learner's progress along the learning curve from *novice* (Score < 60) to *advanced beginner* (Score 60-79), *intermediate* (score 80-99), and *competent* (score 100). The instructor should be able to ascertain, by observing the learner's performance that each of the elements in the tool are covered satisfactorily. (For EBUS-STAT, this could be done once or twice a year in case of learners participating in a subspecialty training program) Repeated testing will demonstrate increases in knowledge and technical skill acquisition as the learner climbs the learning curve from novice to competent bronchoscopist for the procedure being assessed.

To maximize objective scoring, each task has been defined explicitly. Scores can be plotted on a graph, and each institution or program can choose its own cut-offs for a PASS grade, although we recommend that a final PASS grade be achieved with a score of 100, in order for the learner to be judged competent to perform bronchoscopy independently. This is consistent with a philosophy of master training, useful in competency-oriented training. In the absence of a large pilot study demonstrating standard normograms as is done for high-stakes testing, consensus of world renowned experts was obtained to delineate cut-off scores for the following four categories.

Category	Score
Novice	< 60
Advanced Beginner	60-79
Intermediate	80-99
Competent	100

Specific instructions marked by an asterisk (*) are provided in each of the assessment tools.

To administer the EBUS-STAT, learners are asked to perform a complete EBUS-TBNA, while at all times stating what they are doing. Thus, items 1 & 2 assess ability to maneuver the EBUS bronchoscope, item 3 & 6 assesses the ability to obtain a satisfactory image and control the image processor, and items 4, 5, and 7 assess the ability to identify targets, mediastinal anatomy, and perform EBUS-TBNA. Items 8 -10 are scored using the associated quiz images. It is not necessary to test for all the items in the same patient, and some of the EBUS-STAT can be performed using a simulator setting.

EBUS-SAT provides an opportunity for bidirectional feedback that can help identify strengths and weaknesses of individual bronchoscopists, but also of the training program. Ideally, learners should complete the EBUS-SAT prior to the session, providing the completed form to their instructor for consideration and feedback.

EBUS Skills and Tasks Assessment Tool (EBUS-STAT)

ASSESSMENT TOOLS

- Items 1-10 may be scored separately.
- A passing score of 100 is expected to reflect competency.
- Scores >100 should initiate instructor-learner feedback
- Assessments may be performed in models or in patients.
- Knowledge of nomenclature (common language) for EBUS imaging can be assessed using the quiz. Recognition of findings can also be assessed during procedures, in which case instructors may prefer to use the quiz as a learning guide.
- The combined use of the 10 items pertains to technical skills needed to climb the learning curve from novice to competent bronchoscopist able to independently perform EBUS and EBUS-TBNA.
- This assessment tool is complementary to other methods of assessment such as practical approach exercises, checklists, logbooks of numbers of procedures performed, and outcomes.

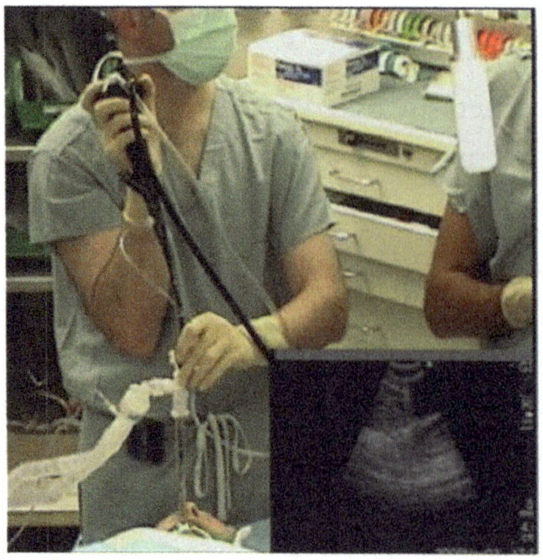

EBUS-STAT 10 Point Assessment Tool

Learner ______________________________ Training Year ________________

Faculty ______________________________ Date ________________________

Educational Item* Items 1-10 each scored separately	Satisfactory Yes/No
1. Able to maneuver the scope through upper airway into trachea, without trauma or difficulty (5 points for single item tested) ☐ Mouth and Vocal cords ☐ ET Tube ☐ Laryngeal mask airway	Yes / No Score _____ /5
2. Able to maneuver scope using white light bronchoscopy within tracheobronchial tree without trauma (4 points, no partial points) ☐ Scope centered in airway lumen avoiding airway wall trauma	Yes / No Score _____ /4
3. Ultrasound image obtained without artifacts (5 points, no partial points) ☐ Absence of artifacts on image, any target	Yes / No Score _____ /5
4. Identify major mediastinal vascular structures (4 points per item) ☐ Aorta ☐ Pulmonary artery ☐ Superior vena cava ☐ Azygos vein ☐ Left atrium	Yes / No Score _____ /20
5. Identify lymph node station (Select 3 targets, 5 points each) ☐ 2R ☐ 2L ☐ 4R ☐ 10R ☐ 7 ☐ 4L ☐ 10L ☐ 11L ☐ 11Rs ☐ 11Ri	Yes / No Score _____ /15
6. Able to operate EBUS processor (2 points each item) ☐ Gain ☐ Depth ☐ Doppler	Yes / No Score _____ /6
7. Performance of EBUS-TBNA (1 point each, target 15 points) ☐ Advance needle through working channel (neutral position) ☐ Secure needle housing by sliding the flange ☐ Release sheath screw ☐ Advance and lock sheath when it touches wall ☐ Release needle screw ☐ Advance needle using jab technique ☐ Visualize needle entering target node ☐ Move stylet in and out a few times ☐ Remove stylet ☐ Attach syringe ☐ Apply suction ☐ Pass needle in and out of node 10-15 times ☐ Release suction ☐ Retract needle into sheath ☐ Unlock and remove needle and sheath	Yes / No Score _____ /15
8. Image analysis: CT scans (1 point each, target 10 points) ☐ Image 1 ☐ Image 2 ☐ Image 3 ☐ Image 4 ☐ Image 5 ☐ Image 6 ☐ Image 7 ☐ Image 8 ☐ Image 9 ☐ Image 10	Yes / No Score _____ /10
9. Image analysis: EBUS views (1 point each, target 10 points) ☐ Image 1 ☐ Image 2 ☐ Image 3 ☐ Image 4 ☐ Image 5 ☐ Image 6 ☐ Image 7 ☐ Image 8 ☐ Image 9 ☐ Image 10	Yes / No Score _____ /10
10. Decision-making tasks: (2 points each, target 10 points) ☐ Image 1 ☐ Image 2 ☐ Image 3 ☐ Image 4 ☐ Image 5	Yes / No Score _____ /10

* The combined use of the 10 items tests competencies needed to climb the learning curve from novice to advanced beginner to intermediate to competent bronchoscopist able to independently perform EBUS-TBNA.

FINAL GRADE PASS FAIL **SCORE** _______/100

EBUS-STAT Questions

NAME ___________________________

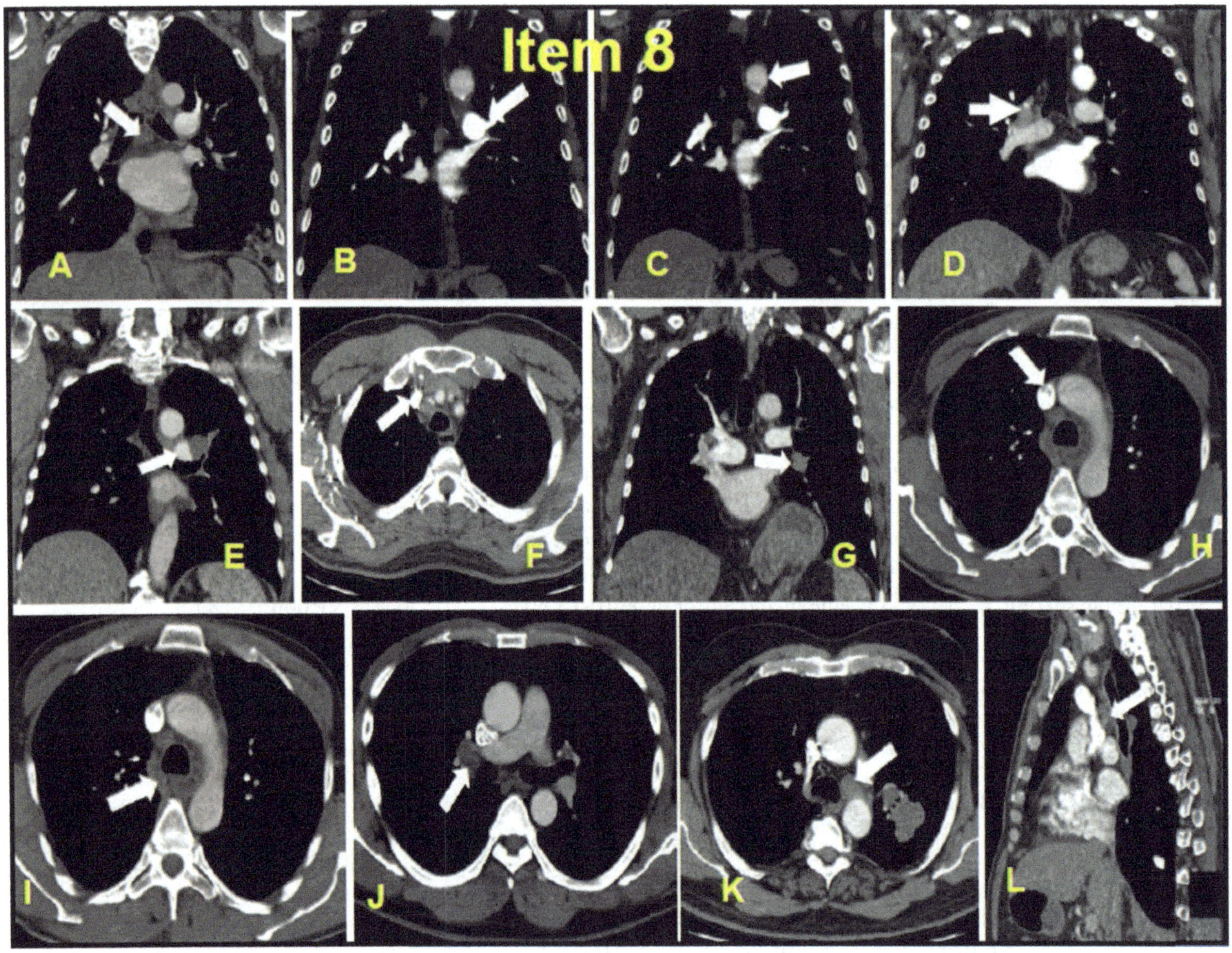

ITEM 8: Match the photo (A-L) to the corresponding 10 CT scan descriptions (Only one response per description)			
____________ Superior vena cava adjacent to 4R	____________ Inominate vein adjacent to 2R	____________ Pulmonary artery adjacent to 4L	____________ Aortic arch adjacent to 4L
____________ Azygos vein adjacent to 4R	____________ Station 7 adjacent to left atrium	____________ Station 11L with adjacent lung	____________ Station 10R
____________ Station 4L in axial view	____________ Pulmonary artery adjacent to 10L	NO RESPONSE	

EBUS-STAT Questions

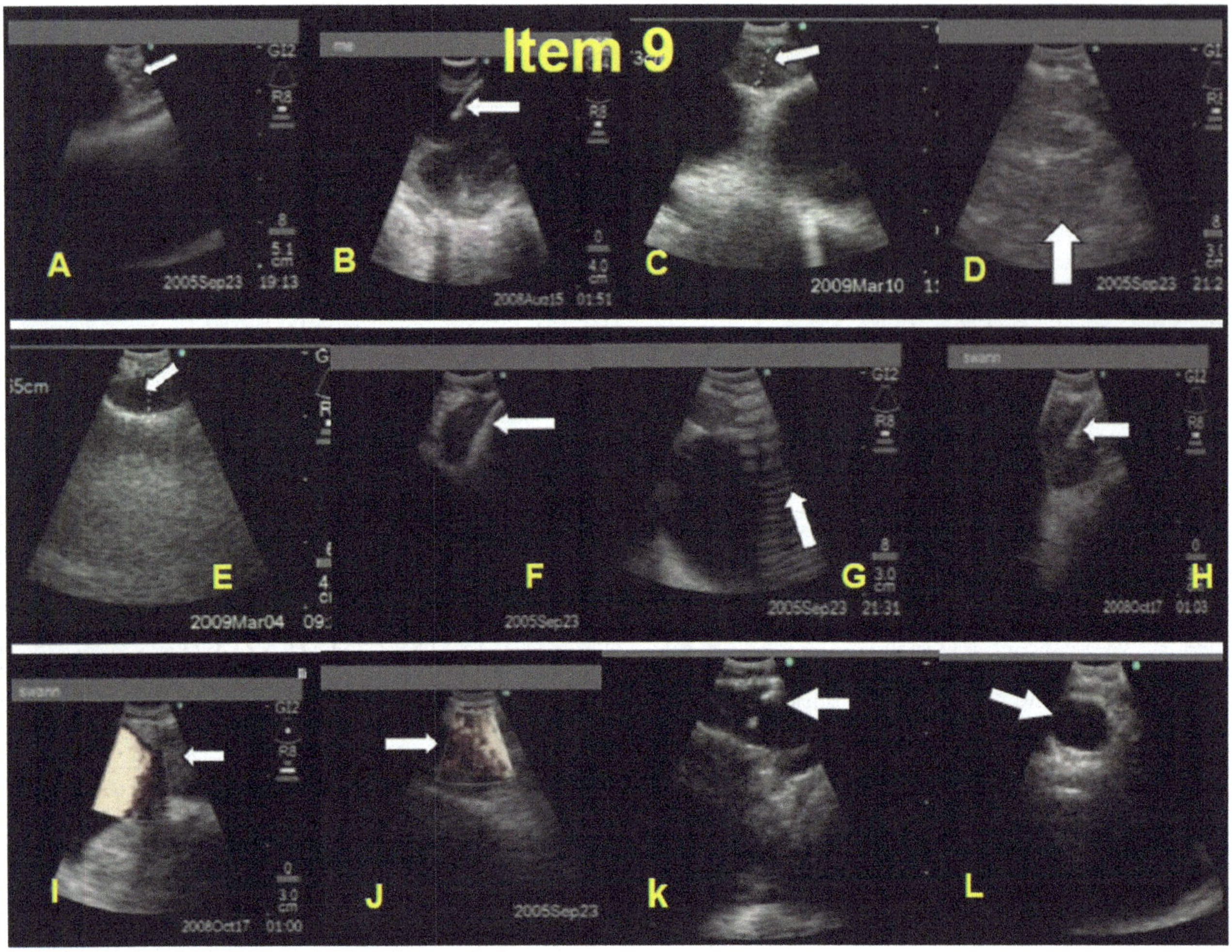

ITEM 9: Match the photo (A-L) to the corresponding 10 EBUS views (Only one response per description)			
________ Station 4R adjacent to pulmonary artery superior vena cava and ascending aorta	________ Needle penetrating through and through	________ Needle missing target node	________ Station 4L adjacent to aorta and pulmonary artery
________ Station 4L adjacent to pulmonary artery	________ Needle within lymph node	________ Normal lung	________ Reverberation artifact
________ Station 7 adjacent to left atrium	________ Hilar node adjacent to normal lung	NO RESPONSE	

ITEM 10: Choose **One** best answer for each question

1. Three FDG avid nodes are noted on Fusion PET-CT in a patient with a Left Upper Lobe PET positive mass. Which node (x, y or z) should be sampled first ?

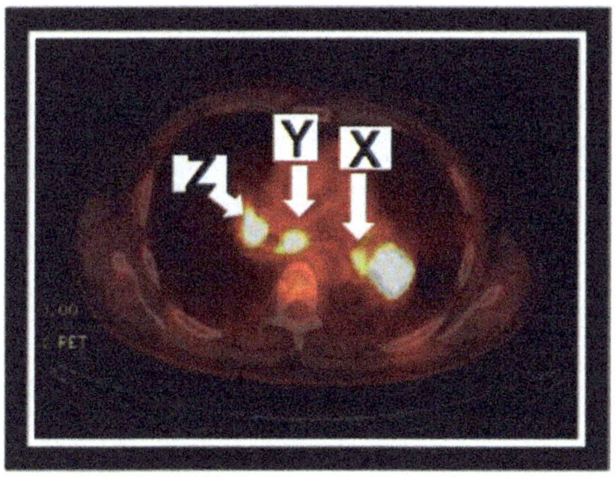

Answer ________

2. Where is the node located (needle insertion site A, B, C, D, E, F,G, or H) using white light bronchoscopy ?

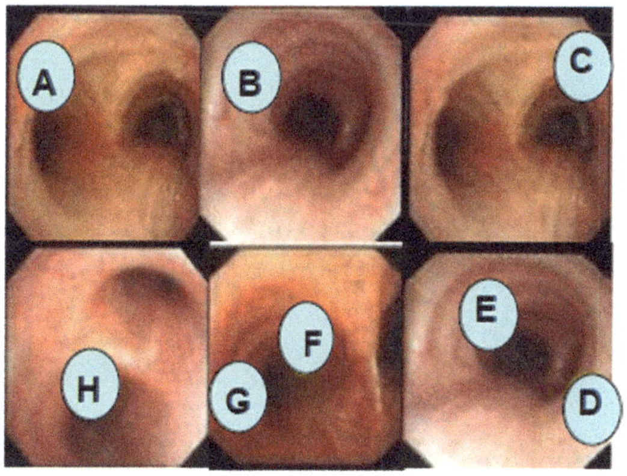

Answer ________

ITEM 10: Choose **One** best answer for each question

3. To sample level 11L, point the scope towards (A), (B), (C)

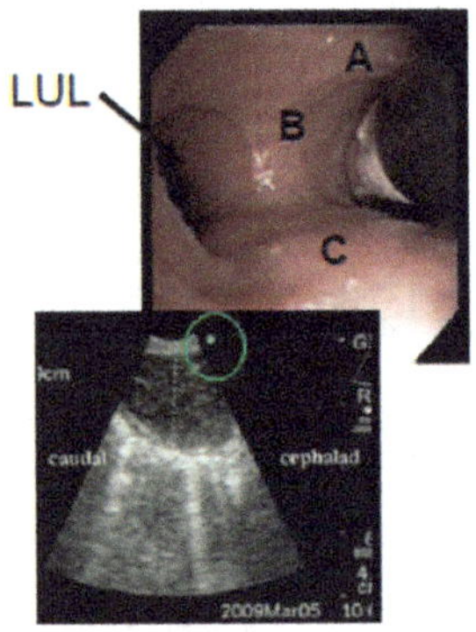

Answer ________

4. When sampling level 4R, consider pointing the scope towards A, B or C).

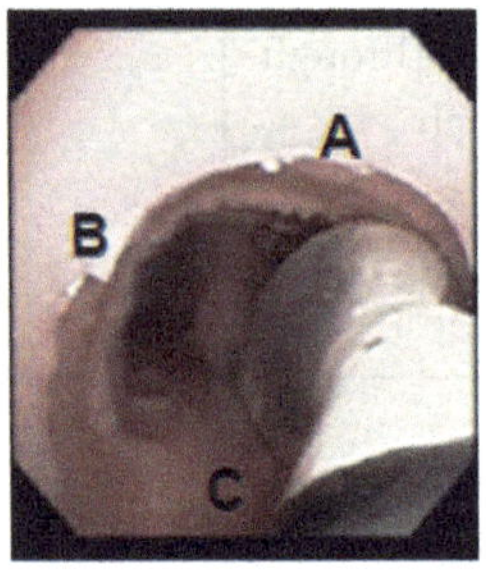

Answer ________

5. The Interlobar Pulmonary Artery is most likely seen when sampling level (A) 10R, (B) 11R, or (C) 12R

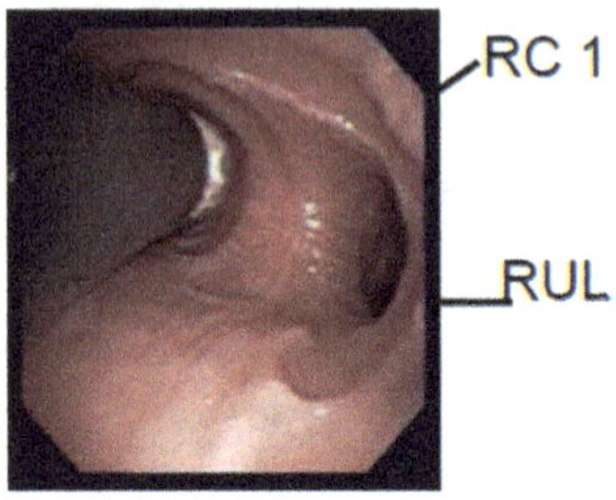

Answer ________

USER INSTRUCTIONS

EBUS-STAT 10 Point Assessment Tool

Learner ______________________________ Training Year ______________

Faculty ______________________________ Date ____________________

Educational Item* Items 1-10 each scored separately	**Satisfactory Yes/No**
1. Able to maneuver the scope through upper airway into trachea, without trauma or difficulty (5 points for single item tested) ☐ Mouth and Vocal cords ☐ ET Tube ☐ Laryngeal mask airway * Educators may wish to "test" only one technique applicable to their institution. This is an "All or None" exercise. No partial points are given. When EBUS-STAT is used as a learning instrument, all THREE techniques should be demonstrated in order to obtain FIVE points.	Yes / No Score ____ /5
2. Able to maneuver scope using white light bronchoscopy within tracheobronchial tree without trauma (4 points, no partial points) ☐ Scope centered in airway lumen avoiding airway wall trauma *The learner should be able to maneuver between lateral and medial walls without traumatizing main and minor carinas.	Yes / No Score ____ /4
3. Ultrasound image obtained without artifacts (5 points, no partial points) ☐ Absence of artifacts on image, any target *Targeting any nodal station, a sharp image without artifacts should be obtained.	Yes / No Score ____/5
4. Identify major mediastinal vascular structures (4 points per item) ☐ Aorta ☐ Pulmonary artery ☐ Superior vena cava ☐ Azygos vein ☐ Left atrium *Each of the vascular structures should be identified on demand. It may be necessary to score this item in several patients.	Yes / No Score ____/20
5. Identify lymph node station (Select 3 targets, 5 points each) ☐ 2R ☐ 2L ☐ 4R ☐ 10R ☐ 7 ☐ 4L ☐ 10L ☐ 11L ☐ 11Rs ☐ 11Ri * Target stations are selected based on indication, anatomy, and instructor preference. To identify all nodal stations, more than one patient may be necessary. In this case, instructors may choose to readminister EBUS-STAT. Stations 2, 4, and 7 can be scored in a low-fidelity model.	Yes / No Score ____/15

6. Able to demonstrate EBUS processor functions (2 points each item) ☐ Gain ☐ Depth ☐ Doppler *Except for Doppler, these functions can be tested in either a low-fidelity model <u>or</u> patient.	Yes / No Score ____/6
7. Performance of EBUS-TBNA (1 point each, target 15 points) ☐ Advance needle through working channel (neutral position) ☐ Secure needle housing by sliding the flange ☐ Release sheath screw ☐ Advance and lock sheath when it touches wall ☐ Release needle screw ☐ Advance needle using jab technique ☐ Visualize needle entering target node ☐ Move stylet in and out a few times ☐ Remove stylet ☐ Attach syringe ☐ Apply suction ☐ Pass needle in and out of node 10-15 times ☐ Release suction ☐ Retract needle into sheath ☐ Unlock and remove needle and sheath *Ideally, while performing EBUS-TBNA, steps should be listed in order by the learner, according to the product manual. As needles and techniques evolve, the steps may change, but principles remain the same to assure equipment, operator, and patient safety, and obtain an adequate specimen.	Yes / No Score ____/15
8. Image analysis: CT scans (1 point each, target 10 points) ☐ Image 1 ☐ Image 2 ☐ Image 3 ☐ Image 4 ☐ Image 5 ☐ Image 6 ☐ Image 7 ☐ Image 8 ☐ Image 9 ☐ Image 10 * This is a written test for which 1 point is given for each correct answer, to be used with associated slide-show or print-out.	Yes / No Score ____/10
9. Image analysis: EBUS views (1 point each, target 10 points) ☐ Image 1 ☐ Image 2 ☐ Image 3 ☐ Image 4 ☐ Image 5 ☐ Image 6 ☐ Image 7 ☐ Image 8 ☐ Image 9 ☐ Image 10 * This is a written test for which 1 point is given for each correct answer, to be used with associated slide-show or print-out.	Yes / No Score ____/10
10. Decision-making tasks: (2 points each, target 10 points) ☐ Image 1 ☐ Image 2 ☐ Image 3 ☐ Image 4 ☐ Image 5 This is a written test for which 2 points are given for each correct answer, to be used with associated slide-show or print-out.	Yes / No Score ____/10

* The combined use of the 10 items tests competencies needed to climb the learning curve from novice to advanced beginner to intermediate to competent bronchoscopist able to independently perform EBUS-TBNA.

FINAL GRADE PASS FAIL **SCORE** ________/100

EBUS Skills and Tasks Quiz Answers

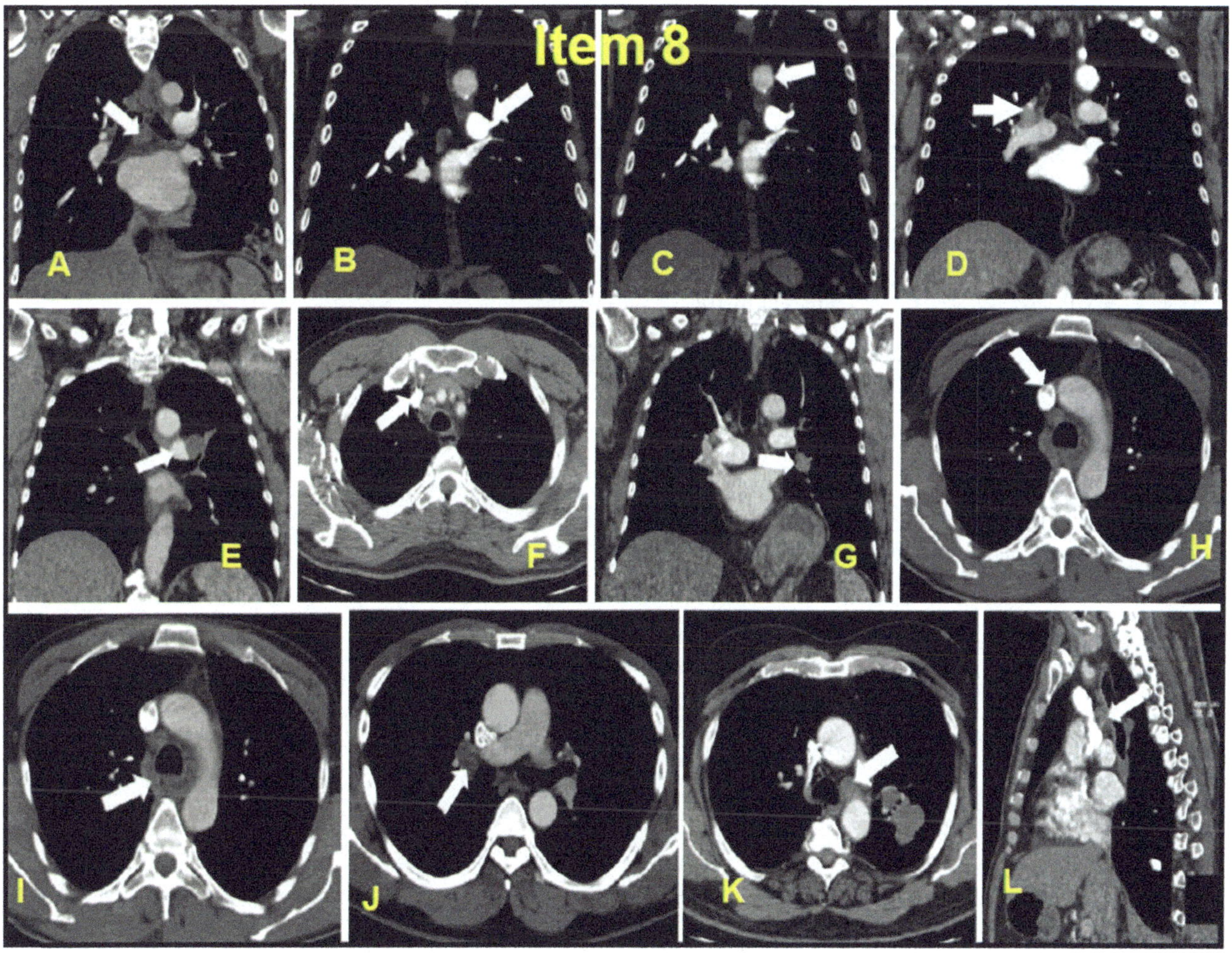

ITEM 8: Match the photo (A-L) to the corresponding 10 CT scan descriptions (Only one response per description)			
H Superior vena cava adjacent to 4R	F Inominate vein adjacent to 2R	B Pulmonary artery adjacent to 4L	C Aortic arch adjacent to 4L
I Azygos vein adjacent to 4R	A Station 7 adjacent to left atrium	G Station 11L with adjacent lung	D Station 10R
K Station 4L in axial view	E Pulmonary artery adjacent to 10L	NO RESPONSE	

EBUS Skills and Tasks Quiz Answers

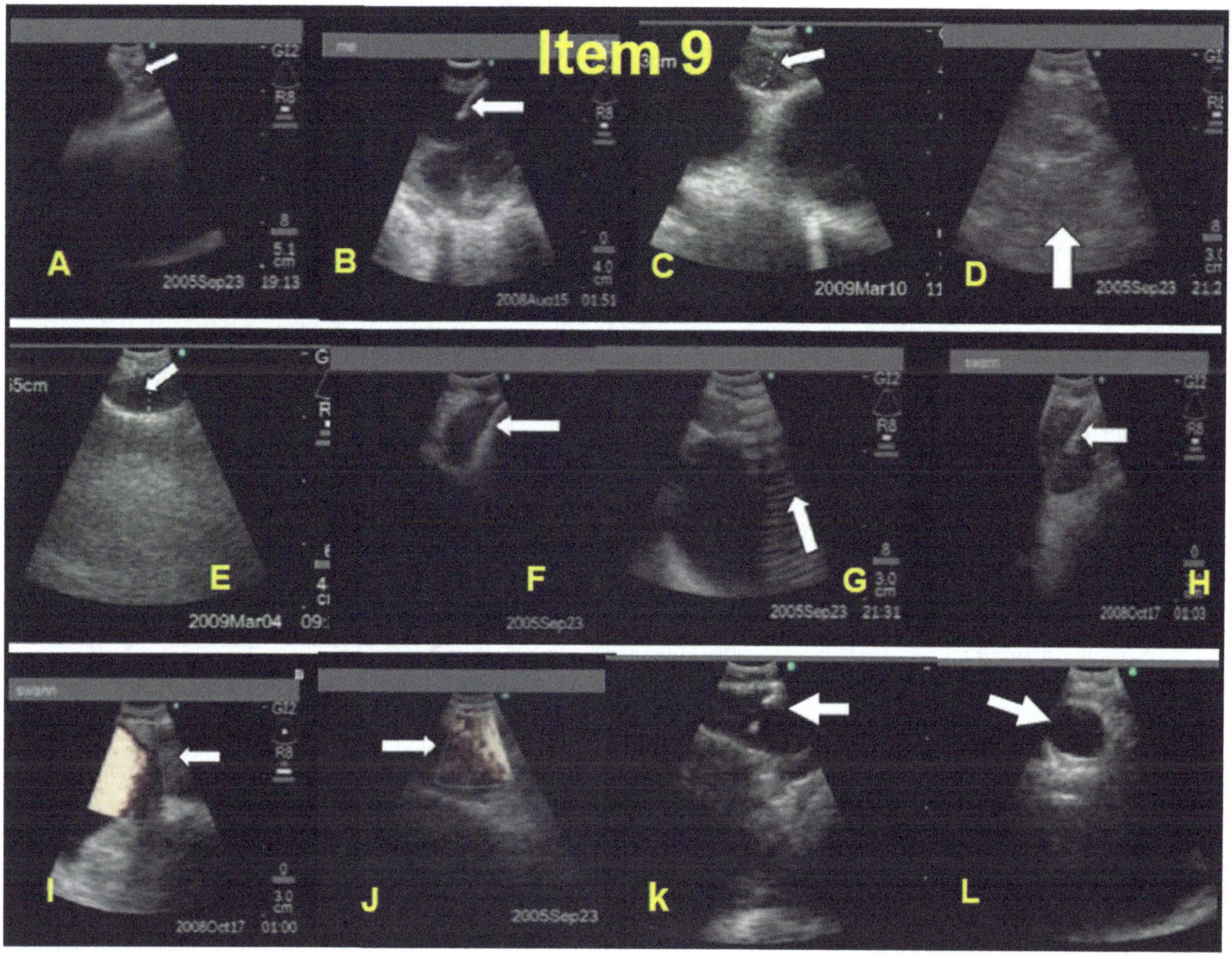

ITEM 9: Match the photo (A-L) to the corresponding 10 EBUS views (Only one response per description)			
A Station 4R adjacent to pulmonary artery superior vena cava and ascending aorta	F Needle penetrating through and through	B Needle missing target node	C Station 4L adjacent to aorta and pulmonary artery
I Station 4L adjacent to pulmonary artery	H Needle within lymph node	D Normal lung	G Reverberation artifact
J Station 7 adjacent to left atrium	E Hilar node adjacent to normal lung	NO RESPONSE	

ITEM 10: Choose **One** best answer for each question

1. Three FDG avid nodes are noted on Fusion PET-CT in a patient with a Left Upper Lobe PET positive mass. Which node (x, y or z) should be sampled first ?	**2.** Where is the node located (needle insertion site A, B, C, D, E, F, G or H) using white light bronchoscopy ?
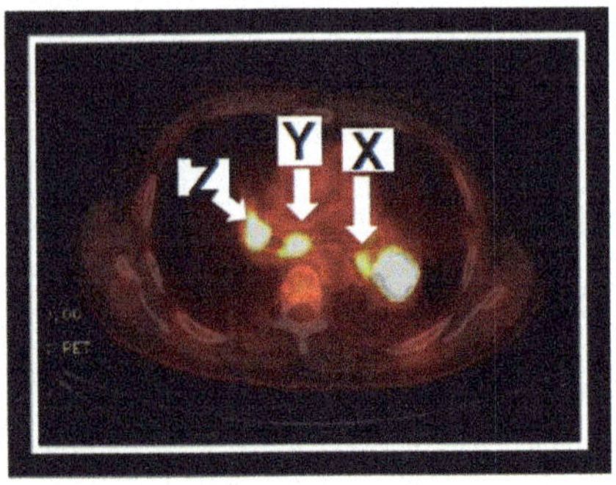	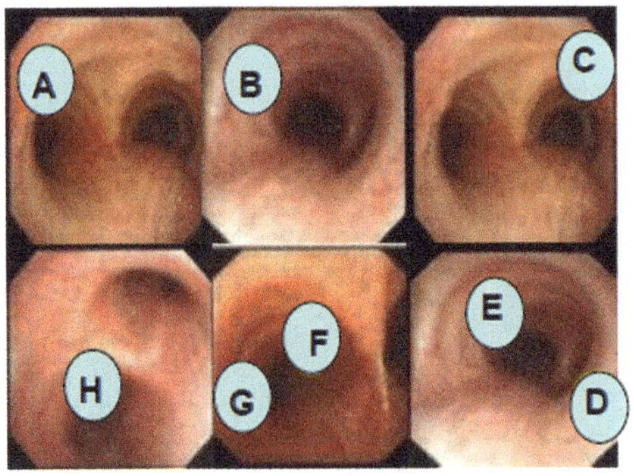
Answer Z	**Answer** H

ITEM 10: Choose **One** best answer for each question

3. To sample level 11L, point the score towards (A), (B), (C).	**4.** When sampling level 4R, consider pointing the scope towards A, B or C).	**5.** The Interlobar Pulmonary Artery is most likely seen when sampling level (A) 10R, (B) 11R, or (C) 12R
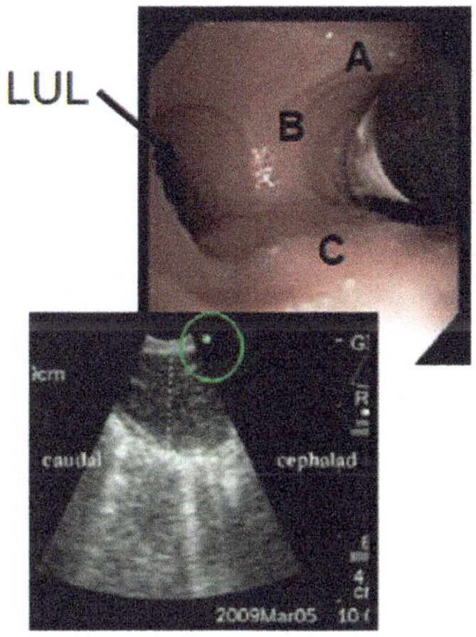	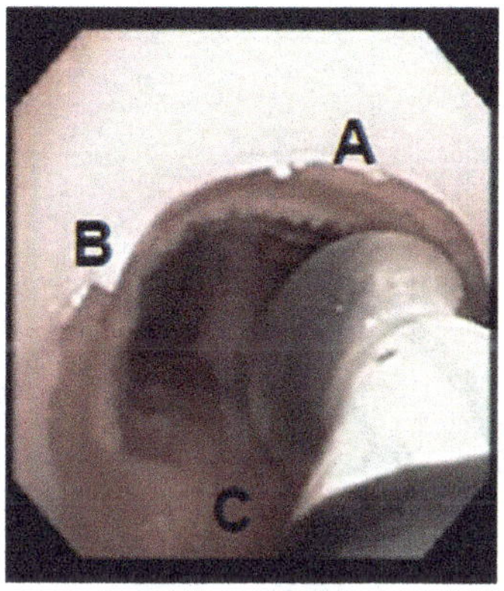	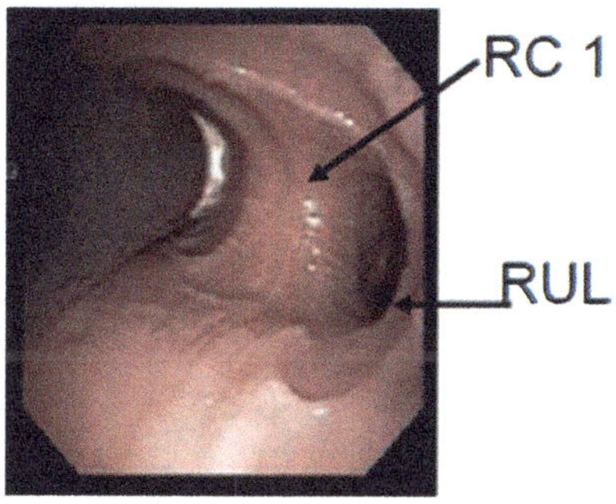
Answer B	**Answer A**	**Answer B**

EBUS Self-Assessment Tool (EBUS-SAT)

- Items 1-10 may be assessed separately.
- There is no "passing score" for this assessment tool.
- The purpose of this assessment tool is to initiate instructor-learner feedback and to identify areas that warrant further reinforcement.
- Assessments may be performed in models or in patients.
- Assessments may be performed before and after a series of training sessions or clinical procedures.
- This assessment tool is complementary to other methods of assessment such as EBUS-STAT, practical approach exercises, checklists, logbooks of numbers of procedures performed, and outcomes.

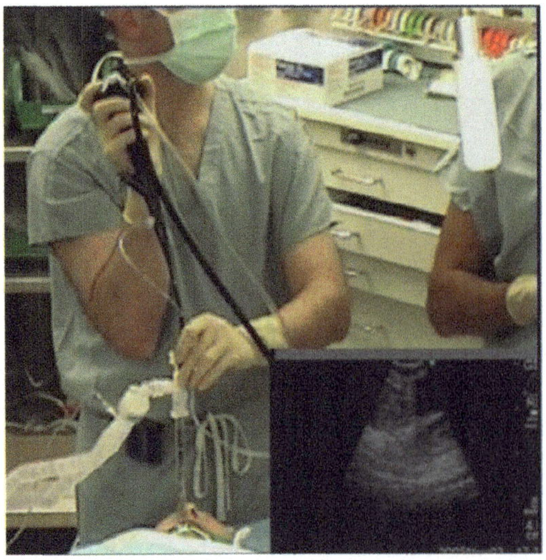

Endobronchial Ultrasound Self Assessment Tool (EBUS-SAT)

The purpose of this assessment tool is to provide bidirectional feedback between learner and instructor. There are no wrong answers. Well performed, this interaction will allow opportunities to ascertain strengths and weaknesses of a training program and educational methodologies. In addition, an open discussion will allow both learner and instructor to identify the learner's zones of proximal development and reflective capacity[1]. Educators may wish to ask learners to complete the EBUS-SAT prior to the encounter, and to then review each element of the questionnaire with the learner in order to identify perceived and real strengths or weaknesses in the performance of various elements of the EBUS-TBNA. Learners should answer each question by writing the number that most closely represents their experience with EBUS and EBUS-TBNA using the following scale.

1	2	3	4	5
Not comfortable		Comfortable		Very comfortable

1.	I am able to introduce the EBUS bronchoscope without difficulty	___
2.	I am able to atraumatically maneuver the EBUS bronchoscope	___
3.	I am able to identify major mediastinal vascular structures	___
4.	I am able to identify lymph node stations 2R and 2L	___
5.	I am able to identify lymph node stations 4R and 10R, 7 and 4L	___
6.	I am able to identify lymph node stations 10L and 11L, 11Rs and 11Ri	___
7.	I am able to use gain, depth and Doppler functions	___
8.	I am able to recognize ultrasound image distortions/artifacts	___
9.	I am able to obtain to obtain an adequate EBUS-TBNA sample	___
10.	I am comfortable independently performing EBUS-TBNA in patients	___

Anatomy Abnormalities Technique Equipment Interpretation of findings

I would like to learn more about (circle all that apply above)

1	2	3	4	5
Poor	Below average	Average	Good	Excellent

Using the above scale please rate this training program as

I have the following comments

[1] The constructivist psychologist Lev Vygotsky (1896-1934) believed that learning and development depend on social interaction. Focusing primarily on how children learn, he described a zone of proximal development (ZPD) as "the distance between the actual development level as determined by independent problem solving and the level of potential development as determined through problem solving under adult guidance or in collaboration with more capable peers" (L.S. Vygotsky: *Mind in Society: Development of Higher Psychological Processes*, p. 86, John-Steiner, Cole, Scribner, and Souberman Editors, Harvard University Press ,1980). Tinsley and Lebak expanded on this theory, describing a zone of reflective capacity in which adults increased their ability for critical reflection through feedback, analyses, and evaluation of one another's work in a collaborative working environment (Lebak, K. & Tinsley, R. Can inquiry and reflection be contagious? Science teachers, students, and action research. Journal of Science Teacher Education;2010:21;953-970).

The Essential EBUS Bronchoscopist©
MODULE 1: Post-test

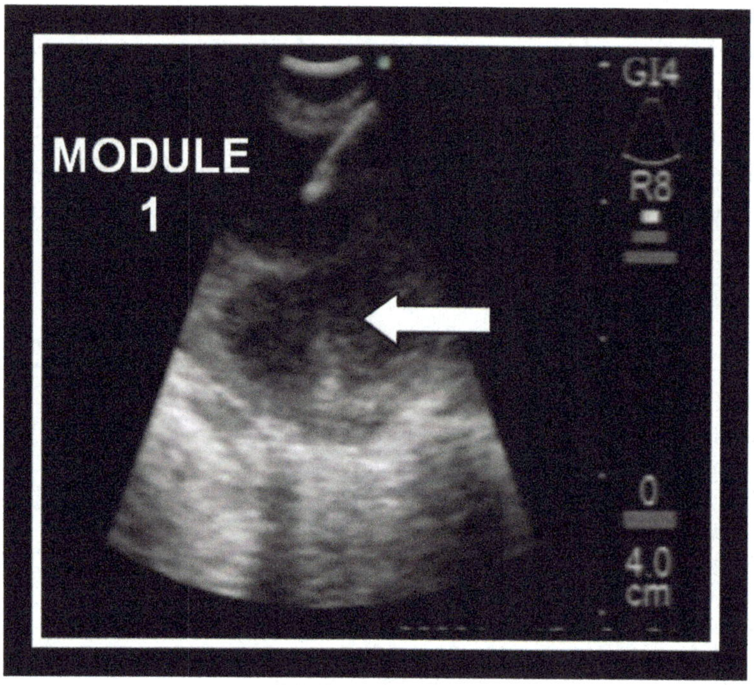

Post-tests are multiple choice, single BEST answer.

While many programs consider 70% correct responses a passing grade, the learner's "target" score should be 100%.

Passing grades are desirable and should be noted on the BEP Program completion checklist.

The Essential EBUS Bronchoscopist© is a single 30 question/answer set with a module-specific competency-oriented list of learning objectives. Information pertains to major topics pertaining to EBUS and convex probe (CP) EBUS-TBNA, including anatomy and ultrasound physics, patient preparation, indications, complications, techniques and solutions to technical difficulties, informed consent, patient safety issues, equipment maintenance, ultrasound imaging patterns, diagnostic yields and expected results. Available on Amazon and from Bronchoscopy.org.

The aim of **The Essential EBUS Bronchoscopist**© is to enhance the learner's progress along the learning curve from novice to competent practitioner. To encourage interactive learning and communication among peers, many question/answer sets are intentionally written so that a correct response is not readily apparent.

Ten post-test questions are best answered after reading the module. None are meant to serve as high stakes tests, but rather as low-stakes continuing self-learning assessments that help document the progressive acquisition of knowledge needed for the safe and competent practice of EBUS and (CP) EBUS-TBNA. Several questions/answer sets of **The Essential EBUS Bronchoscopist**© are used to design validated tests of bronchoscopic knowledge and for didactic lectures or pretest-posttest sessions at regional meetings conducted as part of Bronchoscopy International inspired training sessions. An honor system is assumed in regards to viewing provided answers to these post-tests on the following pages.

The Essential EBUS Bronchoscopist Post test

Please answer the following TEN multiple choice questions. There is a "single" best answer for each question. Your target score is 100% correct responses, although many institutions will use 70% correct responses as a satisfactory grade.

Q1: EBUS TBNA and conventional TBNA are of equal efficacy for sampling which of the following nodal stations?

A. Station 10R
B. Station 4L
C. Station 7
D. Station 5

Q2: Maximum penetration depth of an ultrasound wave depends most on:

A. Frequency
B. Resolution
C. Tissue color
D. Pulse duration

Q3: Representative cytology specimens are best obtained by:

A. Aspirating from the center of the lymph node
B. Noting more than 10% cellularity composed of lymphocytes
C. Repeated aspiration attempts until a tissue core is obtained
D. Aspirating from the periphery of the lymph node

Q4: When the water-filled balloon is not in contact with the airway wall, which of the following artefacts is usually seen?

A. Tadpole tail artefact
B. Comet tail artefact
C. Reverberation artefact
D. Acoustic shadowing

Q5: The typical coagulation necrosis sign seen during EBUS includes which of the following?

A. Hyperechoic area with blood flow
B. Hypoechoic area with blood flow
C. Hypoechoic area without blood flow that sometimes occupies the entire node
D. Hypoechoic area without blood flow, usually in a small section of the node

Q6: In a patient with left upper lobe adenocarcinoma requiring mediastinal staging, which of the following nodal stations should be sampled first?

A. The enlarged, but PET negative contralateral lower paratracheal node
B. The enlarged but PET negative subcarinal node
C. The enlarged ipsilateral PET positive hilar node
D. The enlarged ipsilateral PET positive lower paratracheal node

Q7: Which of the following is an attenuation artefact?

A. The acoustic shadow sign
B. The comet tail sign
C. The pleural reflection sign
D. The hepatization lung sign

Q8: Which of the following is true about lower frequency ultrasound such as that used in EBUS convex probe procedures?

A. Penetration depth is greater than with higher frequency probes
B. Superficial structures are better visualized than with higher frequency probes
C. Airway wall layers are better visualized than with higher frequency probes
D. Resolution is higher than with higher frequency probes

Q9: Laryngeal mask airways (LMA) are helpful while performing EBUS –TBNA because:

A. LMAs can be placed without use of a general anesthetic or hypnotic agent
B. LMAs have a minimal risk of aspiration compared to performing EBUS without an indwelling airway.
C. LMAs facilitate access to level 2 lymph nodes compared to endotracheal tubes.
D. LMAs allow faster awakening compared to performing EBUS with an endotracheal tube.

Q10: Which of the following EBUS-TBNA related complications has the greatest impact on patient management?

A. Inability to sample a level 7 node because of scope breakage during the procedure
B. False negative sampling of a contralateral paratracheal node
C. False negative sampling of an ipsilateral level 10 node
D. Inability to penetrate through the lymph node capsule

EBUS Bronchoscopist© Post-test Answers

ANSWERS TO POST-TEST ANSWERS

1. C	2. A	3. D	4. C	5. C	6. A	7. A	8. A	9. C	10. B

SECTION 10
Checklists

A collection of checklists and user instructions:

- EBUS Sedation-Anesthesia
- EBUS Informed consent
- EBUS Procedural pause
- EBUS Image processor, needle and scope handling
- EBUS Practical Approach
- EBUS Proctored EBUS-TBNA
- EBUS and EBUS-TBNA Program completion

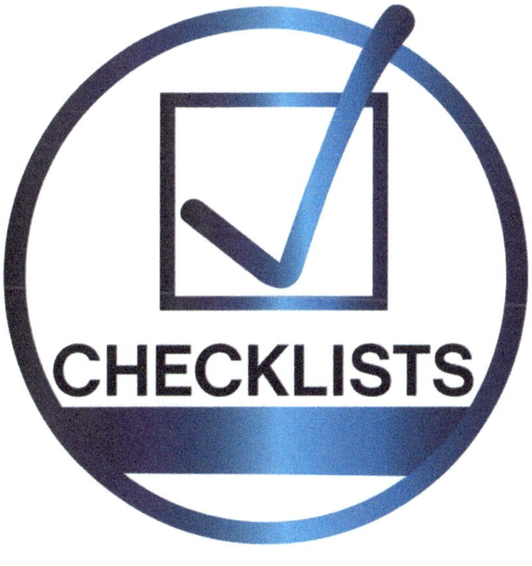

Scoring Recommendations for EBUS CHECKLISTS

(Sedation/Anesthesia, Informed Consent, Procedural Pause, Image Processor, needle and scope handling, Practical Approach, Proctored EBUS-TBNA,)

The goal of these checklists is to be able to monitor a learner's progress along the learning curve from *novice* (Score < 60) to *advanced beginner* (Score 60-79), *intermediate* (score 80-99), and *competent* (score 100). The instructor should be able to ascertain, by observing the learner's performance that each of the TEN elements in each tool are covered satisfactorily. The frequency with which these tools should be used remains to be studied and is currently at the discretion of program directors.

Repeated testing will demonstrate knowledge and skill acquisition as the learner climbs the learning curve from novice to advanced beginner, intermediate and competent bronchoscopist for the procedure being assessed.

To maximize objective scoring, each task in the checklists has been defined explicitly in this user manual. Participation in specially-designed *Train-the-Trainers* courses being currently organized is encouraged to assist with standardization, and to help instructors use this program to its fullest potential.

Scores can be plotted on a graph, and each institution/program can obviously choose its own cut-offs for a PASS grade, although we recommend that a final PASS grade be achieved with a score of 100, in order for the student to be judged competent to perform bronchoscopy independently.

In the absence of a large pilot study demonstrating standard normograms as is done for high-stakes testing, consensus of world renowned experts was obtained to delineate cut-off scores for the following four categories.

Category	Score
Novice	< 60
Advanced Beginner	60-79
Intermediate	80-99
Competent	100

Specific instructions marked by an asterisk (*) are provided in each of the following checklists.

EBUS SEDATION/ANESTHESIA 10-Point CHECKLIST*

Learner ______________________ Training Year ____________

Faculty ______________________ Date ______________

☐ Interactive session ☐ Patient environment

Educational Item* Items 1-10 are scored 10 points each (no partial points given)	**Satisfactory Yes/No**
1. Definitions ☐ Moderate sedation ☐ Deep sedation ☐ General anesthesia	Yes / No
2. Able to obtain sedation-anesthesia informed consent	Yes / No
3. Able to describe ASA classification ☐ 1 ☐ 2 ☐ 3 ☐ 4 ☐ 5	Yes / No
4. Able to identify high risk patients	Yes / No
5. Able to describe potential contraindications	Yes / No
6. Able to list equipment that must be available	Yes / No
7. Sedation/anesthetic agents: role, dosage, precautions ☐ Midazolam ☐ Fentanyl ☐ Propofol	Yes / No
8. Reversal agents: role, dosage, precautions ☐ Flumazenil ☐ Naloxone	Yes / No
9. Able to describe how to respond to complications such as ☐ Vomiting ☐ Seizure ☐ Hypotension	Yes / No
10A. Able to describe how to respond to over-sedation and ☐ Hypotension ☐ Airway obstruction	Yes / No
10B. Able to describe how to respond to over-sedation and ☐ Hypoxemia ☐ Respiratory failure	Yes / No

* Each of the 10 items contains all of the elements required by ACGME (patient care, medical knowledge, practice-based learning and improvement, interpersonal communication skills, professionalism, and systems-based practice).

FINAL GRADE PASS FAIL **SCORE** _______/100

USER INSTRUCTIONS

EBUS Sedation/Anesthesia Checklist

Questions pertaining to sedation can be asked during a separate simulation session or during a patient encounter. The learner will have received the sedation-anesthesia synopsis as well as any institution-specific guidelines and protocols. A passing score of 100, although somewhat subjective, is encouraged.

Educational Item* Items 1-10 are scored 10 points each (no partial points given)	**Satisfactory Yes/No**
1. Definitions ☐ Moderate sedation ☐ Deep sedation ☐ General anesthesia	Yes / No
2. Able to obtain sedation/anesthesia informed consent	Yes / No
3. Able to describe ASA classification ☐ 1 ☐ 2 ☐ 3 ☐ 4 ☐ 5	Yes / No
4. Able to identify high risk patients	Yes / No
5. Able to describe potential contraindications	Yes / No
6. Able to list equipment that must be available	Yes / No
7. Sedation agents: role, dosage, precautions ☐ Midazolam ☐ Fentanyl ☐ Propofol	Yes / No
8. Reversal agents: role, dosage, precautions ☐ Flumazenil ☐ Naloxone	Yes / No
9. Able to describe how to respond to complications such as ☐ Vomiting ☐ Seizure ☐ Hypotension	Yes / No
10A. Able to describe how to respond to over-sedation and ☐ Hypotension ☐ Airway obstruction	Yes / No
10B. Able to describe how to respond to over-sedation and ☐ Hypoxemia ☐ Respiratory failure	Yes / No

* Each of the 10 items contains all of the elements required by ACGME (patient care, medical knowledge, practice-based learning and improvement, interpersonal communication skills, professionalism, and systems-based practice).

FINAL GRADE PASS FAIL **SCORE** _______/100

EBUS INFORMED CONSENT 10-Point CHECKLIST*

Learner ______________________________ Training Year ______________

Faculty ______________________________ Date ______________________

☐ Simulation EBUS-TBNA Workshop ☐ Patient-based EBUS-TBNA Scenario

Educational Item* Items 1-10 are scored 10 points each (no partial points given)	**Satisfactory Yes/No**
1. Able to define "Informed Consent": ☐ Informed decision-making regarding indications and expected outcomes, conflict of interest ☐ Protection from liability ☐ Provides opportunity to assess management strategies ☐ Provides opportunity to discuss risks, benefits, and alternatives	Yes / No
2. Able to discuss diagnosis and pertinent clinical issues	Yes / No
3. Able to describe the purpose of the procedure	Yes / No
4. Able to describe the nature of the procedure	Yes / No
5. Able to describe procedure-related risks	Yes / No
6. Able to describe procedure-related benefits	Yes / No
7. Able to describe alternative procedures regardless of cost ☐ or health care coverage	Yes / No
8. Able to describe potential risks and benefits from ☐ choosing the alternatives	Yes / No
9. Able to describe the risks and benefits of not performing ☐ the procedure or not choosing any of the alternatives	Yes / No
10. Able to demonstrate "effectiveness" of the informed consent process by asking the patient to explain in his or her own words, their understanding of the procedure	Yes / No

* Each of the 10 items contains all of the elements required by ACGME (patient care, medical knowledge, practice-based learning and improvement, interpersonal communication skills, professionalism, and systems-based practice).

FINAL GRADE PASS FAIL **SCORE** _______/100

USER INSTRUCTIONS

EBUS Informed consent Checklist

Educational Item* Items 1-10 are scored 10 points each (no partial points given)
1. Able to define "Informed Consent" ☐ Informed decision-making regarding indications and expected outcomes, conflict of interest ☐ Protection from liability ☐ Provides opportunity to assess management strategies ☐ Provides opportunity to discuss risks, benefits, and alternatives * The instructor may wish that the learner be able to address some of the history of informed consent, and explain how and why informed consent plays a prominent role in medicine today.
2. Able to discuss diagnosis and pertinent clinical issues * Which diagnostic elements and clinical information help guide a patient's choice of procedures? Why is this particular procedure being performed based on diagnosis and clinical issues? This provides the background to the informed consent process and opens the door for a dialogue with the patient so that the patient understands that simple authorization to perform the procedures is not what is being requested.
3. Able to describe the purpose of the procedure * Based on the clinical picture, the procedure is placed into context and the different elements of the procedure (such as to sample lymph nodes, exclude infection, or to diagnose or stage a malignancy) are described.
4. Able to describe the nature of the procedure * The procedure is described in layman's terms.
5. Able to describe procedure-related risks * Risks applicable to the procedure are noted; the learner may offer a few questions and answers, such as when can the patient eat, will the procedure hurt, is there a chance for bleeding, lung collapse, or infection. Some patients may fear death, and so this also may need to be addressed. A description of risks can increase both state and trait anxiety, and therefore, patients should probably be asked about their anxiety level and whether medication or other interventions are desired.
6. Able to describe procedure-related benefits * Benefits should be described clearly, such as diagnosis leads to early treatment, may avoid need for more invasive tests, provide information to other doctors to assist with therapeutic and diagnostic strategies, certain illnesses might be excluded so as to simplify further work-up.

7. Able to describe alternative procedures regardless of cost or health care coverage * Alternatives to EBUS & EBUS-TBNA should be cited and described; these might include, for example, invasive procedures such as open surgery, mediastinoscopy, percutaneous needle aspiration, and noninvasive procedures such as radiographic studies, etc.
8. Able to describe potential risks and benefits from choosing the alternatives * The risks and benefits from each of the alternatives should be addressed and explained. They can be compared to those of EBUS & EBUS-TBNA, and the physician can provide expert opinion as to why EBUS is being proposed and recommended.
9. Able to describe the risks and benefits of not performing the procedure or not choosing any of the alternatives * If EBUS is not performed, the patient should be told about potential consequences, whether or not alternatives are chosen, such as, for example, delayed diagnosis, prolonged illness, endangerment, need for different modes of surveillance or subsequent diagnostic tests or therapeutic measures.
10. Able to demonstrate "effectiveness" of the informed consent process by asking the patient to explain in his or her own words, their understanding of the procedure * The patient should be asked to describe EBUS or EBUS-TBNA and its consequences in general terms. This also provides an opportunity for dialogue.

* Each of the 10 items contains all of the elements required by ACGME (patient care, medical knowledge, practice-based learning and improvement, interpersonal communication skills, professionalism, and systems-based practice).

FINAL GRADE PASS FAIL **SCORE** _______/100

EBUS PROCEDURAL PAUSE 10-Point CHECKLIST*

Learner ______________________ Training Year ____________

Faculty ______________________ Date ______________

☐ Simulation EBUS Workshop ☐ Patient-based EBUS Scenario

Educational Item* Items 1-10 are scored 10 points each (no partial points given)	**Satisfactory Yes/No**
1. Able to define "Procedural Pause" as: ☐ Time-Out ☐ Team communication/patient understanding ☐ Wrong patient, site, procedure ☐ Mandatory in USA	Yes / No
2. Able to describe requirements of the procedural pause: ☐ Immediately before procedure ☐ Correct site, position, procedure ☐ Correct patient ☐ Pertinent medical records and equipment ☐ Verbal acknowledgements by all team members ☐ Elimination of environmental distractions	Yes / No
3. Able to describe the team leader's role	Yes / No
4. Able to describe the nursing team's role	Yes / No
5. Able to describe the patient's role	Yes / No
6. Able to describe other person's roles (technicians, other physicians)	Yes / No
7. Able to list the elements that must be covered: ☐ Patient ☐ Procedure ☐ Side and site ☐ Informed consent ☐ Medical records and equipment ☐ Medications ☐ Allergies/drug reactions ☐ Safety concerns based on history	Yes / No
8. Able to address behaviors in case of distractions	Yes / No
9. Able to describe behaviors in case of disagreements	Yes / No
10. Able to describe other elements pertaining to assuring a culture of safety: ☐ Communication ☐ Ability to prevent and respond to complications ☐ Universal, Droplet, and Airborne pathogen precautions	Yes / No

*Each of the 10 items contains all of the elements required by ACGME (patient care, medical knowledge, practice-based learning and improvement, interpersonal communication skills, professionalism, and systems-based practice).

FINAL GRADE PASS FAIL **SCORE** _______/100

USER INSTRUCTIONS

EBUS Procedural Pause Checklist

1. Able to define "Procedural Pause" as ☐ Time Out ☐ Team communication/patient understanding ☐ Wrong patient, site, procedure ☐ Mandatory in USA
2. Able to describe requirements of the procedural pause ☐ Immediately before procedure ☐ Correct patient ☐ Verbal acknowledgements by all team members ☐ Elimination of environmental distractions ☐ Correct site, position, procedure ☐ Pertinent medical records and equipment
3. Able to describe the team leader's role * Mark the site if applicable, state name, patient, and procedure being performed, lead the time out, assure that all distractions are avoided during the time, requests a new time-out in case distractions occur, assures that time-out is being done according to protocol, addresses discrepancies, cancels procedure if all elements are not ascertained, modifies procedural strategy if applicable according to results of the time out.
4. Able to describe the nursing team's role * Assures patient identification using at least two independent identifiers, assures right side right patient, right procedure, reviews and reads informed consent, assures appropriate medical records and equipment are available, assures appropriate response to complications or adverse events is possible.
5. Able to describe the patient's role *If alert, able to state name, agree with procedure and site, signal family members who might be present.
6. Able to describe other person's roles (technicians other physicians) * Able to state name and role.
7. Able to list the elements that must be covered ☐ Patient ☐ Procedure ☐ Side and site ☐ Informed consent ☐ Medical records and equipment ☐ Medications ☐ Allergies/drug reactions ☐ Safety concerns based on history
8. Able to address behaviors in case of distractions * No one should enter or leave the room during the time-out; any interruptions should prompt renewing the time-out; if a new or second procedure is being performed, time-out should be repeated; individuals should remain silent so that all present can focus on the time-out being performed.

9. Able to describe behaviors in case of disagreements

   * Verbal comments, behavior modification during or after the time-out; anyone should be able to disagree with what is being said during the time-out if it is inconsistent with the informed consent, predesignated procedural strategy, or clinical suspicions.

10. Able to describe other elements pertaining to assuring a culture of safety
    - ☐ Communication
    - ☐ Ability to prevent and respond to complications
    - ☐ Universal, Droplet, and Airborne pathogen precautions

    * It is understood that differences between institutions and countries exist. Guidelines specific to each institution or country of practice can be given to students. General rules and concepts, however, should be understood and are covered in the special simulation session.

EBUS Image Processor, Needle and Scope Handling 10-Point CHECKLIST*

Learner ______________________ Training Year __________

Faculty ______________________ Date ______________

☐ Interactive session ☐ Patient environment

Educational Item* Items 1-10 are scored 10 points each (**no partial points given**)	**Satisfactory Yes/No**
1. Airway access and alternate among EBUS and White light bronchoscopy ☐ Airway access Oral/LMA/ET Tube ☐ Alternate EBUS/WLB	Yes / No
2. Image quality adjustments: **Depth** ☐ Describe ☐ Demonstrate	Yes / No
3. Image quality adjustments: **Gain** ☐ Describe ☐ Demonstrate	Yes / No
4. Image quality adjustments: **Frequency** ☐ Describe ☐ Demonstrate	Yes / No
5. Image quality adjustments: **Doppler** ☐ Describe ☐ Demonstrate	Yes / No
6. Image target measurements: **Cursor placement** ☐ Able to describe cursor placement for measuring lymph node size ☐ Able to demonstrate cursor placement and size measurements	Yes / No
7. Scope: Able to demonstrate balloon placement and functionality for optimal image acquisition ☐ Balloon placement onto scope ☐ Balloon integrity check ☐ Removal of air bubbles	Yes / No
8. Needle: Able to check mechanics and integrity of: ☐ Needle adjuster lock ☐ sheath adjuster knob ☐ Connecting slide	Yes / No
9. Needle: Integrity, retraction, and slider ☐ Integrity ☐ Retracts into sheath ☐ Slider moves freely and locks	Yes / No
10. Needle: Stylet and aspiration syringe integrity and function ☐ Moves freely ☐ Aspiration syringe functions	Yes / No

* Each of the 10 items contains all of the elements required by ACGME (patient care, medical knowledge, practice-based learning and improvement, interpersonal communication skills, professionalism, and systems-based practice).

FINAL GRADE PASS FAIL **SCORE** ______/100

USER INSTRUCTIONS

EBUS Image Processor, Needle and Scope Handling Checklist

Questions pertaining to EBUS can be asked during a separate simulation session or during a patient encounter. The learner will have received the EBUS image processor and needle synopsis as well as any institution-specific guidelines and protocols. A passing score of 100, although somewhat subjective, is encouraged.

Educational Item* Items 1-10 are scored 10 points each (**no partial points given**)	**Satisfactory Yes/No**
1. Able to alternate between EBUS and White light bronchoscopy * The instructor should assure that the operator knows how to switch between white light and EBUS bronchoscopy imaging and screen displays	Yes / No
2. Image quality adjustments: **Depth** ☐ Describe ☐ Demonstrate * The instructor verifies that the learner can describe meaning of depth, and demonstrate depth control on the processor	Yes / No
3. Image quality adjustments: **Gain** ☐ Describe ☐ Demonstrate * The instructor verifies that the learner can describe principles of gain, and demonstrate gain control on the processor	Yes / No
4. Image quality adjustments: **Frequency** ☐ Describe ☐ Demonstrate * The instructor verifies that the learner can describe principles of frequency, and demonstrate frequency control on the processor	Yes / No
5. Image quality adjustments: **Doppler** ☐ Describe ☐ Demonstrate * The instructor verifies that the learner can describe principles of Doppler, and demonstrate Doppler control on the processor	Yes / No
6. Image target measurements: **Cursor placement** ☐ Able to describe cursor placement for measuring lymph node size ☐ Able to demonstrate cursor placement and size measurements	Yes / No

7. Scope: Able to demonstrate balloon placement and functionality for optimal image acquisition ☐ Balloon placement onto scope ☐ Balloon integrity check ☐ Removal of air bubbles * The instructor verifies that the learner can place and troubleshoot balloon-related issues.	Yes / No
8. Needle: Able to check mechanics and integrity of: ☐ Needle adjuster lock ☐ sheath adjuster knob ☐ Connecting slide * The instructor assures that the learned knows how the needle functions (eg. is not bent) and is able to troubleshoot malfunction	Yes / No
9. Needle: Integrity, retraction, and slider ☐ Integrity ☐ Retracts into sheath ☐ Slider moves freely and locks	Yes / No
10. Needle: Stylet and aspiration syringe integrity and function ☐ Moves freely ☐ Aspiration syringe functions * The instructor assures that the learner can verify proper functioning of the stylet and aspiration syringe before performing EBUS-TBNA	Yes / No

* Each of the 10 items contains all of the elements required by ACGME (patient care, medical knowledge, practice-based learning and improvement, interpersonal communication skills, professionalism, and systems-based practice).

FINAL GRADE PASS FAIL **SCORE** _______/100

EBUS PRACTICAL APPROACH 10 Point CHECKLIST*

Learner ______________________ Training Year __________

Faculty ______________________ Date __________

☐ Instructor-learner 30 minute session ☐ Daily rounds & EBUS consultation

Educational Item* Items 1-10 are scored 10 points each (no partial points given)	**Satisfactory Yes/No**
1. Initial evaluation A ☐ Physical examination, laboratory tests, and functional assessment ☐ Comorbidities	Yes / No
2. Initial evaluation B ☐ Support system ☐ Preferences and expectations	Yes / No
3. Procedural strategies A ☐ Indications, contraindications, expected results ☐ Operator and team experience and expertise	Yes / No
4. Procedural strategies B ☐ Risk-benefits and therapeutic alternatives ☐ Informed consent	Yes / No
5. Techniques and results A ☐ Anesthesia and perioperative care ☐ Techniques and instruments	Yes / No
6. Techniques and results B ☐ Anatomic dangers and other risks ☐ Results and complications	Yes / No
7. Long-term management plan A ☐ Outcome assessment ☐ Follow-up tests and procedures	Yes / No
8. Long-term management plan B ☐ Referrals to other specialists ☐ Quality improvement and team evaluation	Yes / No
9. Able to answer case-specific questions ☐ Question 1 ☐ Question 2 ☐ Question 3	Yes / No
10. General ability to provide evidence for and rationally justify decision making ☐ Subjective assessment of learner ability	Yes / No

*These 10 items contains all of the elements required by ACGME (patient care, medical knowledge, practice-based learning and improvement, interpersonal communication skills, professionalism, and systems-based practice).

FINAL GRADE PASS FAIL **SCORE** ______/100

USER INSTRUCTIONS

EBUS Practical Approach Checklist

This practical approach exercise is held as a 30-minute session between learner and instructor, similar to an "oral examination". Of course, programs including Practical Approach-like discussions for each EBUS bronchoscopy consultation may choose to forego a formal session. Using a structured format (the four boxes), learners and instructors are more certain to cover in as great a depth as desired all aspects of a procedure: strategy and planning, techniques and instruments, and response to complications. Because each element is important, items are equally weighted at ten points each with no partial points given. A passing score of 100, although somewhat subjective, is encouraged.

Educational Item* Items 1-10 are scored 10 points each (no partial points given)	**Satisfactory Yes/No**
1. Initial evaluation A ☐ Physical examination, laboratory tests, and functional assessment ☐ Comorbidities	Yes / No
2. Initial evaluation B ☐ Support system ☐ Preferences and expectations	Yes / No
3. Procedural strategies A ☐ Indications, contraindications, expected results ☐ Operator and team experience and expertise	Yes / No
4. Procedural strategies B ☐ Risk-benefits and therapeutic alternatives ☐ Informed consent	Yes / No
5. Techniques and results A ☐ Anesthesia and perioperative care ☐ Techniques and instruments	Yes / No
6. Techniques and results B ☐ Anatomic dangers and other risks ☐ Results and complications	Yes / No
7. Long-term management plan A ☐ Outcome assessment ☐ Follow-up tests and procedures	Yes / No
8. Long-term management plan B ☐ Referrals to other specialists ☐ Quality improvement and team evaluation	Yes / No
9. Able to answer case-specific questions ☐ Question 1 ☐ Question 2 ☐ Question 3	Yes / No
10. General ability to provide evidence for and rationally justify decision making ☐ Subjective assessment of learner ability	Yes / No

*These 10 items contains all of the elements required by ACGME (patient care, medical knowledge, practice-based learning and improvement, interpersonal communication skills, professionalism, and systems-based practice).

FINAL GRADE PASS FAIL **SCORE** _______/100

EBUS PROCTORED EBUS & EBUS-TBNA 10-Point CHECKLIST*

Learner ______________________ Training Year __________

Faculty ______________________ Date ______________

☐ Simulation EBUS Workshop ☐ Patient-based EBUS Scenario

Educational Item* Items 1-10 are scored 10 points each (no partial points given)	**Satisfactory Yes/No**
1. Formulation of effective plan and strategy: ☐ Informed consent obtained, signed and in medical record ☐ History and physical ☐ Review imaging studies ☐ Cost-effective practice ☐ Use of information resources ☐ Applies evidence-based medicine ☐ Use of systems resources	Yes / No
2. Patient safety: ☐ ASA assessment ☐ Airway assessment ☐ Allergies ☐ Medications ☐ Comorbidities	Yes / No
3. Patient safety: ☐ Positioning ☐ Supplemental oxygen ☐ Vital signs ☐ Suction ☐ Bite-block and/or ET tube if applicable ☐ Verifies ability to respond to complications and accessibility of resuscitation equipment	Yes / No
4. Patient and procedural team safety: ☐ Knowledgeable use of image processor ☐ Hand disinfection ☐ Universal precautions ☐ "Time-Out".	Yes / No
5. Procedure: ☐ Premedication ☐ Moderate sedation ☐ Topical anesthetic ☐ General anesthesia as applicable	Yes / No
6. Procedure: ☐ Scope insertion ☐ Empathy and Communication with patient	Yes / No
7. Procedure: ☐ Image processor controls ☐ Balloon attachment and troubleshooting ☐ Needle, stylet, and syringe function and troubleshooting	Yes / No
8. Procedure: ☐ Alternate between white light and EBUS ☐ Image acquisition ☐ Recognition of mediastinal and hilar nodal anatomy ☐ Recognition of mediastinal and hilar vascular structures ☐ Lymph node sampling ☐ Smear preparation and station labeling	Yes / No
9. Communication with staff, patient, and patient family ☐ Puts needs of patient first ☐ Punctuality ☐ Respect ☐ Listening skills ☐ Personal appearance ☐ Initiative & Motivation ☐ Empathy ☐ Honesty ☐ Accepts responsibility	Yes / No
10. Documentation/procedure note ☐ Informative ☐ Accurate ☐ Communication with colleagues	Yes / No

* Each of the 10 items contains all of the elements required by ACGME (patient care, medical knowledge, practice-based learning and improvement, interpersonal communication skills, professionalism, and systems-based practice).

FINAL GRADE PASS FAIL **SCORE** ______/100

USER INSTRUCTIONS

EBUS Proctored EBUS-TBNA Checklist

Educational Item* Items 1-10 each scored 10 points (no partial points given)
1. Formulation of effective plan and strategy ☐ Informed consent obtained, signed and in medical record ☐ History and physical ☐ Review imaging studies ☐ Cost-effective practice ☐ Use of information resources ☐ Applies evidence-based medicine ☐ Use of systems resources * The instructor should be certain that the learner has obtained the informed consent and that it is signed and available. The learner should be able to describe pertinent clinical and radiographic findings and to use evidence-based medicine in addition to any other information gained from other resources, such as faculty expert opinion, advice, and requests by referring physicians, to justify the procedure being performed. The learner should be able to describe the use of institutional resources, and use them according to institutional practices, such as computed tomography, ultrasound, other instruments and equipment. This also includes nursing surveillance, respiratory therapy assistance, on-site cytology, and need for procedure suite, operating theater or intensive care unit. Cost-effectiveness can be discussed in regards to other diagnostic or therapeutic modalities, but also how EBUS bronchoscopy may or may not increase or decrease health-related expenditures in the context of the patient's diagnosis and treatment plan.
2. Patient safety: ☐ ASA assessment ☐ Airway assessment ☐ Allergies ☐ Medications ☐ Comorbidities * ASA and airway assessments should be performed according to the institution's guidelines. Allergies, medications, especially anticoagulants and antiplatelet agents should be noted, comorbidities that might increase the risk of adverse events should also be described and identified.
3. Patient safety: ☐ Positioning ☐ Supplemental oxygen ☐ Vital signs ☐ Suction ☐ Bite-block and/or ET tube, if applicable ☐ Verifies ability to respond to complications and accessibility of resuscitation equipment * These measures should be taken according to institutional biases and protocols.
4. Patient and procedural team safety: ☐ Knowledgeable use of image processor ☐ Hand disinfection ☐ Universal precautions ☐ "Time-Out". * Learners should be observed as they comply with these safety measures. Additional information pertaining to time-out, universal precautions, and knowledge of fluoroscopy are provided in the modules. Protocols may vary among institutions.

5. Procedure:

☐ Premedication ☐ Moderate sedation ☐ Topical anesthetic ☐ General anesthesia as applicable

*These should be administered according to institutional biases and according to protocols.

6. Procedure:

☐ Scope insertion ☐ Empathy and Communication with patient

* Performed according to institutional practices. Empathy and communication with the patient should be observed. Learners should be able to speak comfortably and reassuringly with their patient. Open dialogues should be encouraged to enhance confidence and decrease patient anxiety.

7. Procedure:

☐ Image processor controls ☐ Balloon attachment and troubleshooting

☐ Needle, stylet, and syringe function and troubleshooting

* Performed according to institutional practices.

8. Procedure:

☐ Alternate between white light and EBUS ☐ Image acquisition

☐ Recognition of mediastinal and hilar nodal anatomy ☐ Recognition of mediastinal and hilar vascular structures

☐ Lymph node sampling ☐ Smear preparation and station labeling

* Performed according to institutional practices. It is recognized that not all patients will undergo all of these procedures, therefore, if the institution desires, a different proctored checklist can be completed for each (or each set) of the procedures listed.

9. Communication with staff, patient, and patient family

☐ Puts needs of patient first ☐ Punctuality ☐ Respect

☐ Listening skills ☐ Personal appearance ☐ Initiative & Motivation

☐ Empathy ☐ Honesty ☐ Accepts responsibility

*These are for the most part subjective assessments, and also require feedback from nursing staff. Learners should be told that they will be judged on these items during the course of their training, so that they can obtain feedback from their instructors and improve their performance in these areas.

10. Documentation/procedure note

☐ Informative ☐ Accurate ☐ Communication with colleagues

* Procedure notes may vary according to institution; however, in general, the note should be informative, telling a story about the procedure that referring physicians can understand. The note should be accurate regarding what was done, why it was done, and how it was done. Procedure-related adverse events should be described. Communication with colleagues should be observed, by watching how the learner interacts with the nursing team, other physicians, and with referring physicians. While this element is also, for the most part subjective, in general, communication should be informative, accurate polite, and considerate.

* Each of the 10 items contains all of the elements required by ACGME (patient care, medical knowledge, practice-based learning and improvement, interpersonal communication skills, professionalism, and systems-based practice).

FINAL GRADE PASS FAIL **SCORE** _______/100

Recommendations for using the EBUS and EBUS-TBNA Competency Program Completion Checklist

This checklist contains all of the elements of the EBUS and EBUS-TBNA bronchoscopy curriculum. The purpose of this curriculum is to help learners climb the learning curve from novice and advanced beginner to intermediate then competent EBUS bronchoscopist able to independently perform EBUS and EBUS-TBNA.

This curriculum assures that all learners have completed certain materials to the satisfaction of their instructors. It is understood that some learners may need to repeat certain elements of the curriculum until they obtain a passing grade. Some institutions may wish for their trainees to repeat parts of the curriculum during the course of their training (yearly for example, or during the months prior to completing their training).

Not all learners will progress at the same speed. The frequency with which the checklists and assessments tools are administered is at the discretion of the program or training course directors.

To maximize objective scoring, each element in the program checklist has been defined explicitly in this user manual. Participation in specially-designed *Train-the-Trainers* courses is encouraged to assist with standardization so that instructors may use this program to its fullest potential.

A PASS grade signifies learners have achieved a satisfactory (passing) score in each of the ten elements contained in the curriculum. The overall number of procedures performed by the learner should also be recorded; it is recommended that learners keep a diary-log of their procedures, and that program directors or course instructors conduct feedback sessions with learners to monitor patient-care related outcomes.

****

EBUS and EBUS-TBNA Competency Program Completion Checklist

Educational Item	Complete Yes / No	Assessment Item	Pass/Fail/ Incomplete
1. Participation in regional EBUS course if available*	Yes / No	Post-test scores Target 12/20 (60% correct) Score _______%	Pass / Fail / Incomplete
2. Assigned reading: *The EBUS Bronchoscopist*	Yes / No	Post-test scores Target (70% correct) ____	Pass / Fail / Incomplete
3. Lung cancer staging & lymph node map EBUS-CT-FB correlations EBUS Physics and terminology	Yes / No Yes / No Yes / No	Subjective assessments possible during practical approach exercises or simulation sessions	Pass / Fail / Incomplete
4 Tumor markers synopsis and clinical pathway	Yes / No	Idem	Pass / Fail / Incomplete
5. EBUS Airway access, and image acquisition simulation workshop	Yes / No	Image processor, needle and scope handling 10-pt Checklist : Target 100% Score ______%	Pass / Fail / Incomplete
6. EBUS Airway access and image acquisition patient encounter	Yes / No	Image Processor, Needle & Scope handling 10-pt Checklist: Target 100% Score _______%	Pass / Fail / Incomplete
7. Practical Approach interactive workshop	Yes / No	EBUS Practical Approach 10-pt Checklist: Target 100% Score _______% Subjective Target: Pass	Pass / Fail / Incomplete
8. EBUS-TBNA simulation workshop includes Informed Consent, Patient Safety, Procedural Pause workshops, and EBUS step by step	Yes / No	Target scores 100% EBUS-STAT ______% EBUS-SAT Completed Consider using Informed consent, Procedural Pause, and Processor, needle & scope handling checklists	Pass / Fail / Incomplete
9. EBUS-TBNA Patient encounters	Yes / No	Target scores 100% EBUS-STAT ______% EBUS-SAT completed. May include all checklists	Pass / Fail / Incomplete
10. Proctored case EBUS-TBNA proctored checklist	Yes / No	Proctored EBUS-TBNA 10-pt Checklist: Target 100% Score ______%	Pass / Fail / Incomplete

CONGRATULATIONS

You have now completed

The Endobronchial Ultrasound and EBUS-Guided TBNA Training Manual.

This is an important achievement. We hope this educational experience has been productive and inspiring. In addition to improving your cognitive, affective and experiential knowledge, you have significantly improved your technical skills and your ability to teach others effectively.

Please consider participating in our Faculty Development Programs (Train-the-Trainers) organized by Bronchoscopy International® in collaboration with national and international professional medical societies around the world.

We look forward to receiving your comments regarding our programs

Please do not hesitate to contact your regional organization, or email us at www.bronchoscopy.org

Thank you for participating in **The Bronchoscopy Education Project**!

Made in United States
Orlando, FL
05 November 2026

90208349R00118